AF182499

Potential Therapeutic Strategies for Muscular Dystrophy

Edited by Gisela Gaina

Published in London, United Kingdom

Potential Therapeutic Strategies for Muscular Dystrophy
http://dx.doi.org/10.5772/intechopen.102255
Edited by Gisela Gaina

Contributors
Rituparna Barooah, Amruta Paranjape, Alok Sharma, Hemangi Sane, Nandini Gokulchandran, Zubiya Shaikh, Prerna Badhe, Arjun KM, Purushothaman Senthil, Kandhili Chandrasekaran Gayathri, Saina Swathi, Tomoko Yamamoto, Yukinori Okamura, Ryota Tsukui, Hiromi Onizuka, Kenta Masui, Yoichiro Kato, Gisela Gaina, Ioana Lambrescu, Emilia Manole, Laura Cristina Ceafalan

© The Editor(s) and the Author(s) 2023

The rights of the editor(s) and the author(s) have been asserted in accordance with the Copyright, Designs and Patents Act 1988. All rights to the book as a whole are reserved by INTECHOPEN LIMITED. The book as a whole (compilation) cannot be reproduced, distributed or used for commercial or non-commercial purposes without INTECHOPEN LIMITED's written permission. Enquiries concerning the use of the book should be directed to INTECHOPEN LIMITED rights and permissions department (permissions@intechopen.com).

Violations are liable to prosecution under the governing Copyright Law.

Individual chapters of this publication are distributed under the terms of the Creative Commons Attribution 3.0 Unported License which permits commercial use, distribution and reproduction of the individual chapters, provided the original author(s) and source publication are appropriately acknowledged. If so indicated, certain images may not be included under the Creative Commons license. In such cases users will need to obtain permission from the license holder to reproduce the material. More details and guidelines concerning content reuse and adaptation can be found at http://www.intechopen.com/copyright-policy.html.

Notice

Statements and opinions expressed in the chapters are these of the individual contributors and not necessarily those of the editors or publisher. No responsibility is accepted for the accuracy of information contained in the published chapters. The publisher assumes no responsibility for any damage or injury to persons or property arising out of the use of any materials, instructions, methods or ideas contained in the book.

First published in London, United Kingdom, 2023 by IntechOpen
IntechOpen is the global imprint of INTECHOPEN LIMITED, registered in England and Wales, registration number: 11086078, 5 Princes Gate Court, London, SW7 2QJ, United Kingdom

British Library Cataloguing-in-Publication Data
A catalogue record for this book is available from the British Library

Additional hard and PDF copies can be obtained from orders@intechopen.com

Potential Therapeutic Strategies for Muscular Dystrophy
Edited by Gisela Gaina
p. cm.
Print ISBN 978-1-83768-155-6
Online ISBN 978-1-83768-156-3
eBook (PDF) ISBN 978-1-83768-157-0

We are IntechOpen,
the world's leading publisher of
Open Access books
Built by scientists, for scientists

6,600+
Open access books available

179,000+
International authors and editors

195M+
Downloads

156
Countries delivered to

Our authors are among the
Top 1%
most cited scientists

12.2%
Contributors from top 500 universities

CLARIVATE ANALYTICS
BOOK CITATION INDEX
INDEXED

WEB OF SCIENCE™

Selection of our books indexed in the Book Citation Index
in Web of Science™ Core Collection (BKCI)

Interested in publishing with us?
Contact book.department@intechopen.com

Numbers displayed above are based on latest data collected.
For more information visit www.intechopen.com

For EU product safety concerns:
IN TECH d.o.o., Prolaz Marije Krucifikse Kozulić 3, 51000 Rijeka, Croatia,
info@intechopen.com or visit our website at intechopen.com.

Meet the editor

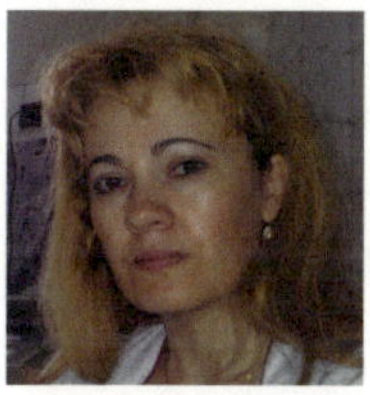

Florina Gisela Gaina, Ph.D., currently works at "Victor Babes" National Institute of Pathology, Bucharest, Romania. She received her Ph.D. in Biology from the University of Bucharest, Romania, in 2009, with a thesis based on the study of the proteins involved in muscular dystrophies. She is a research scientist working in the field of skeletal muscle. The primary focus of her research activities is on skeletal muscle regeneration. Dr. Gaina has been involved in several research projects funded by regional, national, and international public agencies. She is an author and/or co-author of more than twenty scientific papers and conference abstracts and three book chapters.

Contents

Preface **IX**

Chapter 1 **1**
Introductory Chapter: Muscular Dystrophy and Potential Therapeutic Alternatives
by Gisela Gaina

Chapter 2 **5**
Cell Therapy for Muscular Dystrophy
by Alok Sharma, Hemangi Sane, Nandini Gokulchandran, Amruta Paranjape, Zubiya Shaikh, Arjun KM and Prerna Badhe

Chapter 3 **41**
Perspective Chapter: Multiple Functions of *Fukutin*, the Gene Responsible for Fukuyama Congenital Muscular Dystrophy, Especially in the Central Nervous System
by Tomoko Yamamoto, Yukinori Okamura, Ryota Tsukui, Yoichiro Kato, Hiromi Onizuka and Kenta Masui

Chapter 4 **57**
The Potential Benefits of Drug-Repositioning in Muscular Dystrophies
by Ioana Lambrescu, Emilia Manole, Laura Cristina Ceafalan and Gisela Gaina

Chapter 5 **81**
Advanced Physiotherapy Intervention for Muscular Dystrophy
by Saina Swathi, Kandhili Chandrasekaran Gayathri and Purushothaman Senthil

Chapter 6 **95**
Role of Applied Physiology in Management of Muscular Dystrophy by Yoga and Meditation
by Rituparna Barooah

Preface

Muscular dystrophy (MD) is an encompassing term that pertains to a cluster of hereditary neuromuscular disorders. These disorders are distinguished by the gradual deterioration of muscle strength, which arises from diverse mutations in different genes responsible for standard muscle structure and function.

Despite significant advancements in the molecular characterization and diagnosis of MD in recent years, most forms still lack effective treatment. Consequently, the management and rehabilitation of patients remains crucial in maintaining an acceptable level of functional ability. Therefore, research priorities have been and continue to be the development of various efficacious therapeutic options aimed at decelerating the progression of the disease and enhancing the quality of life and lifespan of individuals affected by it.

The present publication offers a comprehensive examination of recent progress in muscle illnesses, encompassing various topics about the genetic underpinnings of multiple forms of MD, potential therapeutic interventions, and the advantages associated with repurposing drugs for treating these conditions.

Also, this book analyzes the impact of different types of exercise training as adjunct therapies in mitigating problems, decelerating pathophysiological progression, and enhancing overall quality of life. It should be mentioned that the effects of exercise on the condition have yet to be comprehensively elucidated. However, recent studies have demonstrated that engaging in appropriate forms of physical activity can enhance the muscular strength of those with MD.

The knowledge and ideas presented within its pages will serve as a source of inspiration for both young and experienced researchers, enabling them to address the numerous inquiries that arise in the field of muscle pathology.

I want to thank all the authors who contributed to this book. I also want to thank Publishing Process Manager Ms. Kristina Kardum Cvitan at IntechOpen for her patience and valuable advice throughout the preparation of this book.

Gisela Gaina
Cell Biology,
Neurosciences and Experimental Myology Laboratory,
Victor Babes Institute of Pathology,
Bucharest, Romania

Chapter 1

Introductory Chapter: Muscular Dystrophy and Potential Therapeutic Alternatives

Gisela Gaina

1. Introduction

Muscle disorders, known as myopathies, are rare or extremely rare diseases that may be classified into two categories: inherited and acquired. The inherited ones include illnesses caused by X-linked, autosomal-recessive, or autosomal-dominant inheritance patterns in distinct genes-encoding proteins that play critical roles in muscle form and function. Different mutations that can occur in these genes alter the function of the proteins responsible for muscle structural support and homeostasis and lead to diseases with different degrees of severity. Duchenne muscular dystrophy (DMD), with the allelic form Becker muscular dystrophy (BMD), is the most frequent and severe form of muscular dystrophy (MD) that affects children, followed by myotonic dystrophy (DM1) and facioscapulohumeral muscular dystrophy (FSHD). Despite advances in understanding MD mechanisms and the development of molecular investigative techniques, no effective treatment is currently available. Over the past two decades, research efforts have focused on characterizing disease mechanisms and developing various diagnostic tools for muscular dystrophy and inherited disorders that affect skeletal and cardiac muscle tissues and are characterized by progressive muscle weakness, wasting, and muscle degeneration. At the same time, research was also directed toward improving the quality of life and life expectancy of patients affected by these diseases by developing promising experimental strategies.

2. Potential therapeutic alternatives for muscular dystrophies

Despite differences in causation and symptoms, nearly all types of muscular dystrophy induce muscle weakness and loss, leading to limits in everyday activities and fatigue [1]. Thus, the researches were oriented to slow the progression of symptoms and ameliorate various kinds of muscular dystrophy through exercise-based therapies [2], pharmacological approaches oriented both targeting the primary defect and the downstream pathological changes [3], cell-based therapy and gene therapy treatments aimed to correct the genetic mutations. Among therapies targeting the primary genetic defect, exon-skipping is one the most promising therapeutic strategies. The most research and the most valuable results were obtained in the studies on DMD [4], the most common form of muscular dystrophy with fatal outcomes. In DMD patients, some mutations in the *DMD* gene change the reading frame and lead to the production of a nonfunctional protein—dystrophin. Exon skipping approaches use antisense oligonucleotides (ASOs) to alter transcript splicing to modulate protein expression. Thus, an out-of-frame mutation becomes an in-frame mutation, the reading frame is restored, and a partially functional dystrophin protein can be produced. A severe DMD phenotype is thus transformed into a milder BMD phenotype, which results in a later onset of symptoms, a slower rate of disease progression [5], and implicitly, a higher life expectancy.

With progress in ASO chemistry, reduced toxicity, and increased potency, exon-skipping approaches have also been developed for other muscular conditions such as dysferlinopathy [6], sarcoglycanopathies [7], laminopathies [8] as well as for other diseases like cancer [9, 10], Parkinson disease [11], and rheumatoid arthritis [12]. However, this approach is estimated to be costly and needs lifelong administration.

In the last period, gene editing with CRISPR/Cas9 (clustered regularly interspaced short palindromic repeats/Cas9) has rapidly become the most widely used tool for editing allowing more precise gene editing [13] and is a promising therapeutic that can permanently correct a mutation. Despite recent developments, restrictions such as delivery efficiency remain. Nevertheless, additional research is needed to ensure the CRISPR system's safety and precision before it can be used in clinical trials.

Another interesting approach for muscular dystrophy, known as repurposing, uses existing drugs that are already approved for use and have been tested in humans for various other diseases [14]. Prior knowledge of information about their pharmacology, pharmacokinetics, and potential toxicity is particularly important for people with life-threatening illnesses, such as MDs, who cannot wait for a traditional medicine development cycle. This urgent need for new therapeutic options for these severe diseases means that drug repositioning could be a possible answer.

In conclusion, this book covers some distinctive aspects of these pathologies and potential therapies and palliative care to improve muscle function.

Author details

Gisela Gaina
Cell Biology, Neurosciences and Experimental Myology Laboratory, Victor Babes Institute of Pathology, Bucharest, Romania

*Address all correspondence to: gisela.gaina@ivb.ro

IntechOpen

© 2023 The Author(s). Licensee IntechOpen. This chapter is distributed under the terms of the Creative Commons Attribution License (http://creativecommons.org/licenses/by/3.0), which permits unrestricted use, distribution, and reproduction in any medium, provided the original work is properly cited.

References

[1] Emery AE. The muscular dystrophies. Lancet. 2002;**359**(9307):687-695 [Internet] Available from: https://linkinghub.elsevier.com/retrieve/pii/S0140673602078157

[2] Gianola S, Castellini G, Pecoraro V, Monticone M, Banfi G, Moja L. Effect of Muscular Exercise on Patients with Muscular Dystrophy: A Systematic Review and Meta-Analysis of the Literature. Front Neurol. Nov 12 2020;**11**:958. DOI: 10.3389/fneur.2020.00958

[3] Guiraud S, Davies KE. Pharmacological advances for treatment in Duchenne muscular dystrophy. Current Opinion in Pharmacology. 2017;**34**:36-48 [Internet] Available from: https://linkinghub.elsevier.com/retrieve/pii/S147148921630100X

[4] Aartsma-Rus A, Fokkema I, Verschuuren J, Ginjaar I, van Deutekom J, van Ommen G-J, et al. Theoretic applicability of antisense-mediated exon skipping for Duchenne muscular dystrophy mutations. Human Mutation. 2009;**30**(3):293-299 [Internet] Available from: https://onlinelibrary.wiley.com/doi/10.1002/humu.20918

[5] Mercuri E, Bönnemann CG, Muntoni F. Muscular dystrophies. Lancet. 2019;**394**(10213):2025-2038 [Internet] Available from: https://linkinghub.elsevier.com/retrieve/pii/S0140673619329101

[6] Aartsma-Rus A, Singh KHK, Fokkema IFAC, Ginjaar IB, van Ommen G-J, den Dunnen JT, et al. Therapeutic exon skipping for dysferlinopathies? European Journal of Human Genetics. 2010;**18**(8):889-894 [Internet] Available from: http://www.nature.com/articles/ejhg20104

[7] Aartsma-Rus A. Overview on AON Design. 2012. pp. 117-29. Available from: https://link.springer.com/10.1007/978-1-61779-767-5_8

[8] Scharner J, Figeac N, Ellis JA, Zammit PS. Ameliorating pathogenesis by removing an exon containing a missense mutation: A potential exon-skipping therapy for laminopathies. Gene Therapy. 2015;**22**(6):503-515 [Internet] Available from: https://www.nature.com/articles/gt20158

[9] Luna Velez MV, da Silva P, Filho O, Verhaegh GW, Hooij O, El Boujnouni N, et al. Delivery of antisense oligonucleotides for splice-correction of androgen receptor pre-mRNA in castration-resistant prostate cancer models using cell-penetrating peptides. The Prostate. 2022;**82**(6):657-665 [Internet] Available from: https://onlinelibrary.wiley.com/doi/10.1002/pros.24309

[10] Dewaele M, Tabaglio T, Willekens K, Bezzi M, Teo SX, Low DHP, et al. Antisense oligonucleotide–mediated MDM4 exon 6 skipping impairs tumor growth. The Journal of Clinical Investigation. 2015;**126**(1):68-84 [Internet] Available from: https://www.jci.org/articles/view/82534

[11] Cole TA, Zhao H, Collier TJ, Sandoval I, Sortwell CE, Steece-Collier K, et al. α-Synuclein antisense oligonucleotides as a disease-modifying therapy for Parkinson's disease. JCI Insight. 2021 Mar 8;**6**(5):e135633. DOI: 10.1172/jci.insight.135633

[12] Yilmaz-Elis S, Aartsma-Rus A, Vroon A, van Deutekom J, de Kimpe S, tHoen PAC, et al. Antisense oligonucleotide mediated exon skipping as a potential strategy for the treatment

of a variety of inflammatory diseases such as rheumatoid arthritis. Annals of the Rheumatic Diseases. 2012;**71** (Suppl. 2):i75-i77 [Internet] Available from: https://ard.bmj.com/lookup/doi/10.1136/annrheumdis-2011-200971

[13] Mali P, Yang L, Esvelt KM, Aach J, Guell M, DiCarlo JE, et al. RNA-guided human genome engineering via Cas9. Science (80-). 2013;**339**(6121):823-826 [Internet] Available from: https://www.sciencemag.org/lookup/doi/10.1126/science.1232033

[14] Vitiello L, Marabita M, Sorato E, Nogara L, Forestan G, Mouly V, et al. Drug Repurposing for Duchenne Muscular Dystrophy: The Monoamine Oxidase B Inhibitor Safinamide Ameliorates the Pathological Phenotype in mdx Mice and in Myogenic Cultures from DMD Patients. Front Physiol. Aug 14 2018;**9**:1087. DOI: 10.3389/fphys.2018.01087

Chapter 2

Cell Therapy for Muscular Dystrophy

Alok Sharma, Hemangi Sane, Nandini Gokulchandran, Amruta Paranjape, Zubiya Shaikh, Arjun KM and Prerna Badhe

Abstract

Muscular dystrophy is a major unmet medical need associated with an inevitable progressive muscle damage and loss of function. Currently, treatment is only symptomatic and supportive. This chapter focuses on cell therapy as a potential treatment approach for muscular dystrophy. Mechanism of action of cell therapy and its ability to alter disease pathology have been discussed. A review of preclinical and clinical studies has been presented with the advantages and shortcomings of various cell types. Rationale for our treatment protocol and experience of treating muscular dystrophy patients has been discussed. Our published results have shown the efficacy of the intrathecal and intramuscular administration of autologous bone marrow mononuclear cells in different types of muscular dystrophy patients. The scores on outcome measures such as 6-minute walk distance, North star ambulatory assessment, Brooke and Vignose scale, Functional independence measure, and manual muscle testing either improved or were maintained suggestive of slowing down disease progression. Efficacy and safety of the treatment was also studied using comparative MRI-MSK and EMG showing decreased fatty infiltration in various muscles post-cellular therapy. Thus, it was found that autologous BMMNC transplantation is a safe and effective treatment option and improves the quality of life of MD patients.

Keywords: muscular dystrophy, stem cells, cell therapy, autologous, bone marrow mononuclear cells

1. Introduction

The term 'muscular dystrophy' first used by Erb (1891), is used for a heterogeneous group of disorders that are hereditary in nature and are characterized by primary involvement of muscles and a tendency for progressive muscle weakness and wasting [1]. They are inherited as X-linked, autosomal dominant, or recessive disease. Over 30 variants of muscular dystrophy (MD) have been identified using genetic or histochemical testing [2, 3]. Most commonly found types of MDs are Duchenne Muscular Dystrophy

(DMD), Becker Muscular Dystrophy (BMD), Limb Girdle Muscular Dystrophy (LGMD), Emery-Dreifuss Muscular Dystrophy (EDMD), Fascioscapulohumeral Muscular Dystrophy (FSHMD), Oculopharyngeal Muscular Dystrophy (OPMD), and Congenital Muscular Dystrophy (CMD). The overall worldwide prevalence of combined MDs is estimated to be 3.6 per 100,000 individuals [4].

Although the onset of symptoms and the rate at which disease progresses is variable and depends mainly on the gene mutation [5], MD is associated with an inevitable progressive muscle damage and loss of function. Loss of ambulation, contractures and deformities are common. Scoliosis is frequently seen in wheelchair-dependent patients. Although the disorder primarily affects skeletal muscles, structural and functional abnormalities are also known to be seen in cardiac muscle, smooth muscle, and the brain [6–8]. Impairment of respiratory function due to weakness of the respiratory muscles is frequent. Cardiac involvement is a feature commonly seen in DMD, BMD, myotonic dystrophy, LGMD, EDMD and CMD. Functional involvement of the brain has also been seen in CMD, myotonic dystrophy, DMD and in some LGMD variants. About one-third boys with DMD have co-morbid mental retardation and other behavioral or psychiatric comorbidities [9, 10].

Currently, treatment is mainly symptomatic and supportive. Though corticosteroids delay loss of function, it is ineffective in stopping progression in MDs. Steroids only reduce inflammation and long-term use is associated with side effects including stunted growth, cataracts, and osteoporosis [11]. MDs represent a major unmet medical need and are associated with progressive disability causing economic and personal burden. Many of the MDs result from mutations in the genes encoding components of the dystrophin-glycoprotein complex (DGC) [12] that links the extracellular matrix of muscle fiber with the F-actin cytoskeleton. The DGC plays an important role in providing mechanical support to the plasma membrane during muscle fiber contraction and is thought to protect muscle fibers from contraction induced damage [13, 14]. Its disruption leads to altered mechanical and signaling functions resulting in increased entry of calcium, immune cell infiltration, progressive muscle wasting, necrosis, and membrane fragility (**Figure 1**) [15, 16]. Gene therapy using viral and non-viral vectors can be a promising treatment option for MD but shows adverse immune responses to vectors raising concerns regarding safety of the treatment [17]. Antisense oligonucleotide (ASO) mediated exon skipping therapy is also a treatment option for MD which targets removal of introns from pre-mRNA to give functional proteins. Currently ASOs for mutations in dystrophin gene amenable to exons 51,53 and 45 are approved by Food and Drug Administration (FDA) which showed the resumption of dystrophin production in MD patients. But the expense of ASOs, its off-target effects and its delivery are current concerns regarding their use [18].

Although the initial cause of muscle damage is genetic in origin, there is now increasing evidence of stem cell dysfunction in MD [19–21], as a contributing factor to the progression of the disease. Blau et al. reported a defect in the proliferative capacity of resident stem cells in DMD [19]. Also, there is increased inflammatory responses in MD patients that disrupt muscle homeostasis and inhibit muscle repair and regeneration [22–24]. It is observed that in DMD and several other forms of MD, the regenerated muscles are prone to degeneration, producing repeated cycles of degeneration and regeneration. As a result, the resident stem cell population is either exhausted or loses the potential to mediate repair leading to progressive replacement of muscle tissue with adipose and fibrotic tissue [25]. Therefore, gene therapy alone

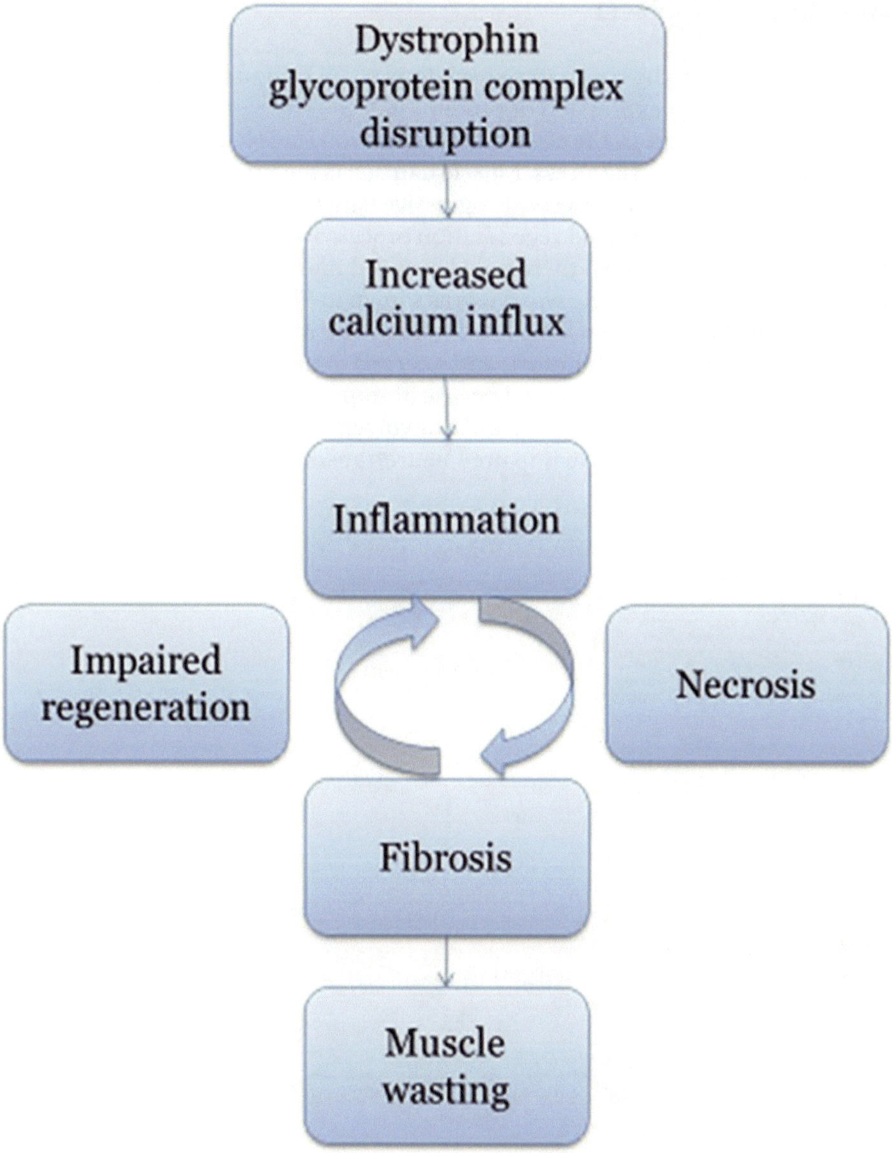

Figure 1.
Sequelae of DGC disruption in MD.

is inadequate as it cannot replenish the stem cell pool and even where applicable and available clinically, needs to be combined with treatment approaches that replenish the stem cell pool.

The objective of any effective treatment lies in restoring dystrophin expression in muscle fibers and in promoting regeneration of muscle fibers. While dystrophin restoration can be achieved by gene therapy or cell therapy or combination of the two, regeneration of muscle can be achieved through cell therapy only and it, therefore, represents an essential treatment approach for MDs.

2. Pathophysiology of MD

As described earlier, the core pathophysiology of MD (**Figure 2**) is genetic mutations resulting in altered expression of proteins in DGC and stem cell dysfunction. DGC is the essential component of the cell wall; its alteration leads to increased cell damage even with minimal contractile stress. Muscle damage is repaired by resident muscle stem cells also known as satellite cells. Progressive damage of the muscle is repaired with continuous satellite cell mediated regeneration process which leads to depletion in the satellite cells pool. Due to which there is an increased muscle damage leading to adipose tissue infiltration causing muscle weakness as shown in **Figure 3** [26]. Increased damage also increases the immune cell infiltration resulting in increased inflammation [27]. Inflammation accelerates cell apoptosis and necrosis in the damaged areas [28]. Also, in MD the muscle function is affected because of impaired blood supply to the muscle leading to chronic ischemia. The DGC is also involved in the formation of synaptic connectivity, abnormal DGC leads to impaired neurotransmission and abnormally formed

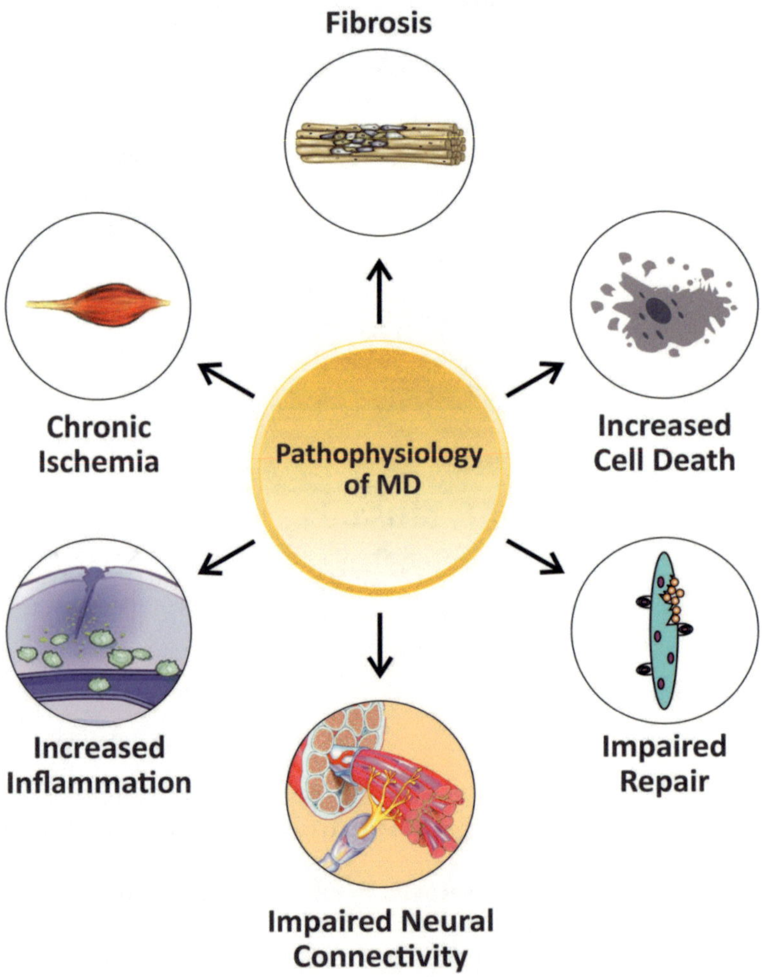

Figure 2.
Pathophysiology of MD.

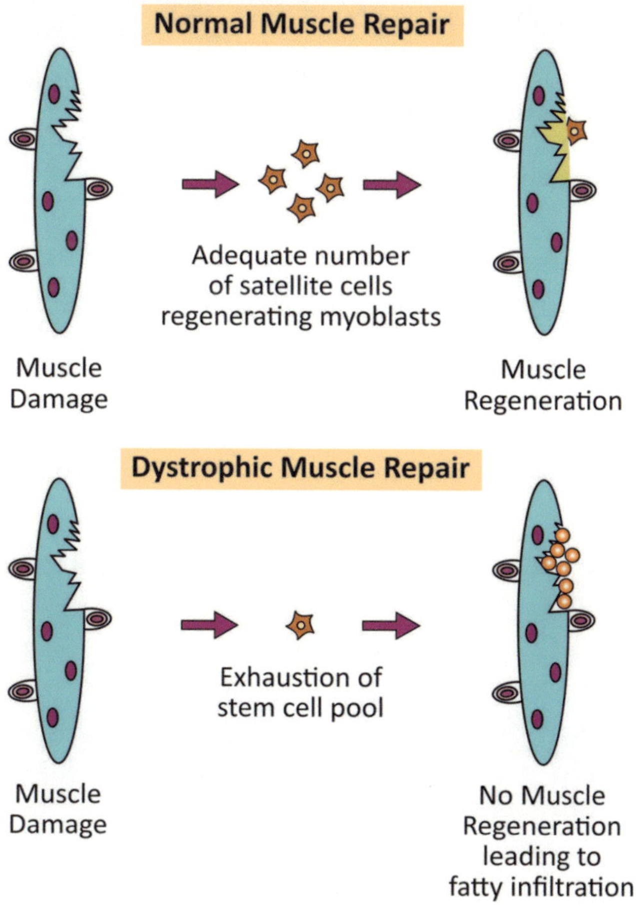

Figure 3.
Normal muscle repair having adequate number of satellite cells versus dystrophic muscle repair demonstrating exhaustion of stem cells.

neural junctions increasing muscle wasting [29, 30]. Hence, the pathophysiology of MD is Multifaceted having multiple contributing factors.

3. Role of stem cells in MD

Stem cells have the ability of self-renewal and migration to the site of damage/ injury and carry out repair and restoration processes. They divide and differentiate to replace the damaged and dead cells [31]. In Vitro experiments have shown that stem cells restore dystrophin expression in duchenne-skeletal muscle cells [32]. Stem cells halt further damage by exerting paracrine mechanisms and stimulate endogenous cells to carry out repair processes. Stem cells secrete various cytokines and chemokines exerting anti-inflammatory, anti-apoptotic, angiogenic and immune-modulatory effects [33]. Effectiveness of cell therapy depends on various factors such as number of cells, route of delivery, myogenic potential, migration and homing capabilities of cells, type of MD and extent of muscle damage. Cell therapy can be a promising long-term solution for MD [34].

4. Understanding stem cells

Stem cells are unique undifferentiated cells characterized by their ability for self-renewal and for differentiation into specialized cell lineages [35].

4.1 Classification of stem cells

4.1.1 Based on potency

Stem cells can be classified according to their ability to differentiate as (**Figure 4**):

- *Totipotent stem cells* that can differentiate to form any tissue including entire organism;
- *Pluripotent stem cells* that can differentiate to all tissue types but not to an entire organism;
- *Multipotent stem cells* that can differentiate into multiple cell types but within one organ system only;

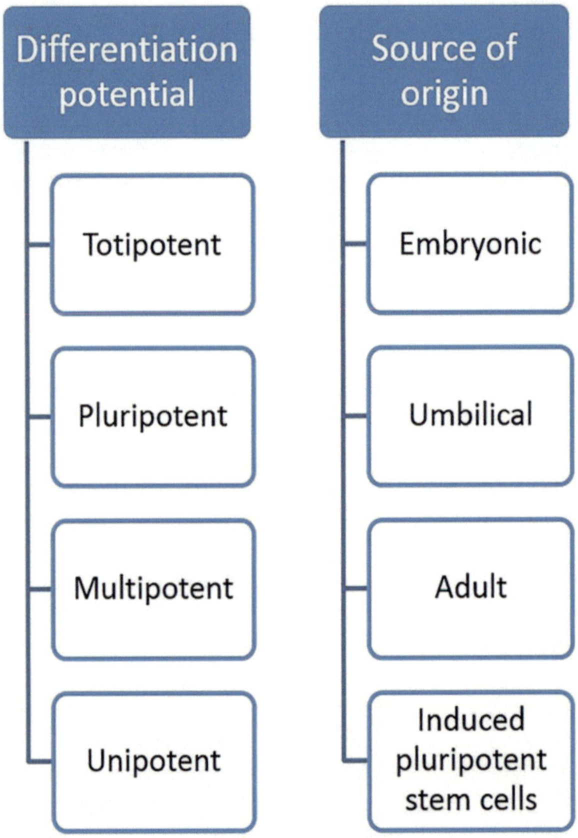

Figure 4.
Classification of stem cells.

- *Unipotent stem cells* are highly specialized stem cells that can differentiate into one cell type committed to a single lineage [36].

4.1.2 Based on their source

Depending on the source, they can be differentiated (**Figure 4**) into

- Embryonic stem cells (ESCs) are pluripotent stem cells derived from inner cell mass of blastocysts.
- Umbilical cord stem cells can be easily derived from umbilical cord without any risk to the donor.
- Adult stem cells are multipotent cells and can be derived from bone marrow, adipose tissue etc.
- Induced pluripotent stem cells (iPSCs) are produced by reprogramming differentiated multipotent adult stem cells to the pluripotent state that can differentiate into any cell of the organism.

Human ESCs are faced with ethical considerations and are also associated with a risk of tumorigenicity whereas umbilical cord stem cells and adult stem cells do not possess ethical concerns.

Cells procured from the patients themselves are autologous cells. Stem cells acquired from donors are allogenic cells. Autologous cells are safer than allogenic cell as they do not show immune rejection while proper HLA typing of donor and recipient is required in case of allogenic cells.

5. Cell therapy as a therapeutic strategy for MD

5.1 Preclinical evidence of effectiveness of cell therapy in MD

5.1.1 Induced pluripotent stem cells

Therapeutic use of ESCs is restricted due to immune rejection and ethical concerns. These concerns have however been overcome partly by Yamanaka et al. by showing that iPSCs can be generated from somatic cells [37]. Pre-clinical studies have shown the ability of myoblasts and mesenchymal stem cells (MSCs) derived from iPSCs to fuse with mature muscle fibers [38, 39] and improve muscle function in dystrophic mice [40].

5.1.2 Stem cells of muscle tissues

Another type of cell that is Myoblast cells, naturally residing in the muscles, are the primary skeletal muscle stem cells responsible for maintenance of resident stem cell pool by self-renewal and repair of adult skeletal muscle and were the source of stem cells in the earliest cell-based therapies for treating MDs [41]. Pre-clinical studies demonstrated that myoblasts can be expanded in vitro [42, 43] and are able to regenerate muscle [44–46]. Stem cells other than myoblasts that are present within muscle and possess myogenic potential include muscle derived stem cells [47–49], mesoangioblasts [50–52], muscle derived stem cells, pericytes, CD 133+ stem cells and muscle side population cells that can contribute to muscle regeneration [53]. Transplantation of allogenic muscle derived stem cells contributed to muscle repair, dystrophin expression, satellite cell replenishment and clinical efficacy in MD dogs [54]. Recently, mesoangioblasts, pericytes and CD 133+ have demonstrated promise as stem cell source in treatment of MDs due to their ability to contribute to muscle regeneration and because they can be delivered systemically. Also, mesoangioblasts can reconstitute the satellite cell pool [55]. The ability of mesoangioblasts to contribute to muscle regeneration and to restore muscle structure and function has been tested in the mouse model of LGMD [56, 57] and in the dog model of DMD [58]. Tedesco et al. demonstrated expression of normal dystrophin in muscle fibers and production of functional muscle fibers in mice model of DMD following intramuscular injection of genetically corrected mesoangioblasts [55]. However, the disadvantage of these cell types is their limited ability to colonize in the muscles due to incomplete adhesion and extravasation of these cells [52, 56]. Pericytes are known to be developmentally derived from mesoangioblasts [50, 59], possess myogenic potential and have shown to promote muscle regeneration in dystrophic mice following intra-arterial delivery [59, 60]. Though promising, further research of the role of mesoangioblasts and pericytes in muscle regeneration are required. Torrente et al. demonstrated that CD 133+ cells contributed to muscle regeneration in dystrophic mice [61]. These cells can migrate through blood vessel walls [62]. Intramuscular and intra-arterial application of genetically corrected CD 133+ cells resulted in significant improvement in muscle function and dystrophin expression in dystrophic mice [63]. Laumonier et al. showed that Pax7+/MyoD− muscle reserve stem cells of human origin in immunodeficient mice intramuscularly promoted lacerated muscle regeneration [64].

5.1.3 Bone marrow derived stem cells

Furthermore, Hematopoietic stem cells (HSCs) and MSCs are the two main cell types that can be isolated from the adult bone marrow. MSCs are multipotent stem cells and possess the ability to differentiate into myoblasts [65]. Additionally, MSCs can induce an anti-inflammatory effect and anti-apoptosis through paracrine function. These cells can be easily isolated from the bone marrow, are relatively safe and have minimal tumorigenicity. Ferrari et al. demonstrated that marrow derived stem cells can migrate to areas of degeneration and participate in muscle regeneration [66]. Intravenous delivery of bone marrow stem cells in the mouse model of DMD, donor derived nuclei were incorporated into muscle with partial restoration of dystrophin expression [67]. Maeda et al. showed intraperitoneal transplantation of bone marrow derived MSCs in DKO (dystrophin-utrophin double-knockout) mice increased satellite cells in mice, improved their locomotion, reduced kyphosis, and increased their longevity [68].

5.1.4 Wharton jelly derived stem cells

Park et al. demonstrated that intravenous transplantation of human Wharton jelly derived MSC regenerated muscles, reduced apoptosis, and fibrosis in mdx mice model [69].

5.2 Clinical evidence

Only myoblasts, bone marrow derived stem cells and to a lesser extent umbilical cord-MSCs, muscle derived CD 133+ and cardiosphere derived stem cells (CDCs) have been investigated in humans.

Though safety and dystrophin production were seen in a case of DMD following myoblast transplantation [70], dystrophin production was seen in some but not all the later studies [71–80]. Although clinical benefit was observed in many studies, clinical use of these cells is hindered by several disadvantages. They cannot be delivered to all the muscles via systemic route, expansion in culture reduces their regenerative capacity [81], allogenic transplantation requires immunosuppression, and these cells have poor dispersion after intramuscular injection [82]. Also, these cells fail to participate in long term regeneration [83] and rapidly die in the first 72 hours after transplantation [84]. These problems have been tried to be resolved [85], but interest in use of these cells in treatment of MD has waned.

There is an ongoing Phase I/II clinical trial using systemic transfer of allogenic muscle derived mesoangioblasts from HLA identical donors in DMD [86]. Autologous transplantation of muscle derived CD 133+ cells in 8 boys with DMD was found to be safe and demonstrated an increased capillary per muscle fiber ratio with a switch from slow to fast myosin-positive myofibers [87]. 82 patients with progressive MD received double transplantation of autologous bone marrow derived MSCs and umbilical cord MSCs [88]. Treatment efficacy was evident in 68 of the 82 patients with no adverse event during the treatment course. Intravenous transplantation of allogenic cord blood cells in a patient with DMD resulted in improved function in standing, walking, and turning over with a mild graft versus host disease (GVHD) [89]. In another study, umbilical cord derived MSCs intravenously and intramuscularly in 11 DMD patients caused stabilization of muscle power as compared with control group and demonstrated safety without inducing GVHD [90]. A total of 15 studies demonstrated the benefits of intrathecal and intramuscular autologous bone marrow mononuclear cell transplantation in MD [91–105]. Dai et al. demonstrated four times administration of allogenic Wharton jelly-derived MSCs via intra-arterial and intramuscular routes in 9 DMD patients resulted in improved pulmonary function and increased dystrophin level with no adverse effects [106]. Another study revealed that intramuscular transplantation of fetal progenitor cells in 22 DMD patients improved their muscle activity, gait quality and reduced pseudohypertrophy [107]. The safety and efficacy of intravenous administration of human allogenic CDCs was studied by Mcdonald et al. in 26 late stage-DMD patients in a multicentre, randomized, double-blind, placebo-controlled, phase 2 clinical trial. The patients showed improved cardiac function and structure with maintained upper limb function with no major adverse effects [108].

6. Our experience of autologous bone marrow mononuclear cell therapy in MD treatment

6.1 Our treatment protocol

After careful review of available literature and evidence, we have a protocol that we follow for stem cell transplantation at NeuroGen Brain and Spine Institute.

6.1.1 Patient selection

The patient's selection is based on the World Medical Association's Helsinki declaration of Ethical Principles for medical research involving human subjects. The protocol was reviewed by the Institutional Ethics Committee (IEC) which is registered with the Central Drugs Standard Control Organization (CDSCO).

6.1.2 Pre-intervention evaluation

Before cell therapy intervention, the patients undergo a comprehensive evaluation consisting of neurological examination as well as evaluation on various outcome measures such as 6-minute walk distance, North star ambulatory assessment, Brooke and Vignose scale, Functional independence measure and manual muscle testing (MMT). Motor points of the patients are also identified and plotted for the weak muscles by experienced physiotherapists in which BMMNCs are to be injected.

6.1.3 Transplantation of BMMNCs

Transplantation of autologous bone marrow mononuclear cells intrathecally and intramuscularly is done in 3 steps (**Figure 5**). The protocol includes 300mcg granulocyte colony-stimulating factor (GCSF) administration subcutaneously 48 hours and 24 hours before cell therapy to enhance mobilization of cells [109]. 80–120 ml of bone marrow is aspirated from the anterior superior iliac spine. Mononuclear cells are then separated using the density gradient method. The separated cells are checked for viability under microscope using trypan blue and CD34+ cells are identified using fluorescence-activated cell sorting (FACS) analysis. Separated cells are then transplanted intrathecally and intramuscularly. The cells are diluted in the patient's own cerebrospinal fluid and divided into two parts. One part is transplanted intrathecally by lumbar puncture at the level between 4th and 5th lumbar vertebrae and the other part is further divided and injected intramuscularly at the motor point of muscles that are weak and of functional importance. Motor point is the point at which the innervating nerve enters a muscle, and it has the highest density of myoneural junctions. The

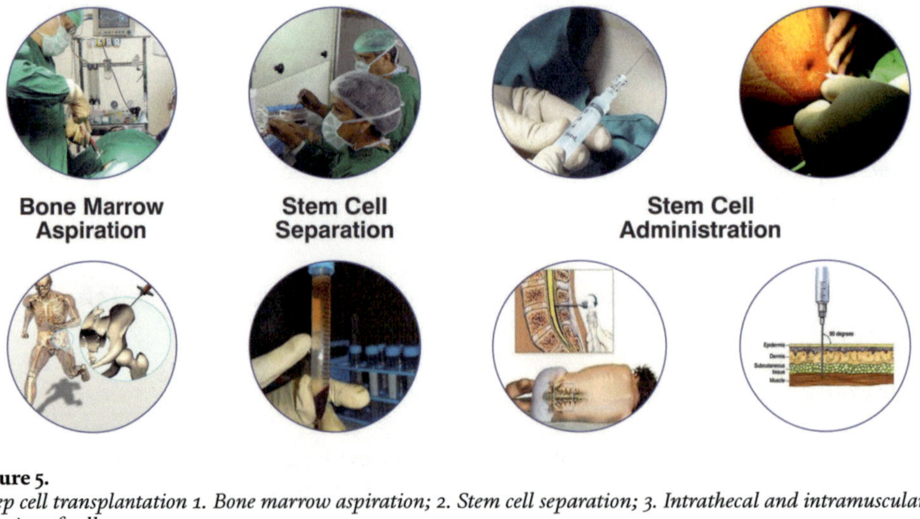

Figure 5.
3 step cell transplantation 1. Bone marrow aspiration; 2. Stem cell separation; 3. Intrathecal and intramuscular injection of cell.

identification of motor points is made by using electrical stimulation. A motor point can be identified as a superficial point overlying a muscle that exhibits a contraction at lowest level of stimulation (faradic stimulation with pulse duration of 1 millisecond).

6.1.4 Neurorehabilitation

The transplantation is followed with an individualized rehabilitation program incorporating physiotherapy, occupational therapy, speech therapy, aquatic therapy, psychological counseling, and dietary and nutritional advice. Patients are closely monitored for post procedure adverse events during their hospital stay. They are advised to continue the rehabilitation program at home preferably under professional supervision after discharge.

6.1.5 GCSF administration

After cell therapy, patients are also given one GCSF injection per month for the next 6 month after cell therapy that mobilizes the stem cells and improves muscle strength in MD patients [110, 111].

6.1.6 Follow up and adverse event monitoring

Patients are monitored for short term adverse reactions during their 4 days hospital stay. Patients are also advised to have regular follow-up at 3 months and 6 months, followed by yearly follow-up. During each follow-up, the patients undergo complete neurological assessment and are monitored for any long-term adverse effects.

6.2 Rationale for the protocol

6.2.1 Autologous bone marrow mononuclear cells

Although autologous bone marrow mononuclear cells carry the genetic abnormality in patients of MD, they have shown the potential to alter disease pathology and thereby disease progression. Also, autologous cell transplantation is not faced with the risk of immune rejection and therefore does not need immunosuppression. Bone marrow derived cells are easy to isolate, are excluded from ethical concerns, can be easily accessed, and transplanted [112], sufficient number of cells can be obtained by minimally invasive procedure and are marked by no immunogenicity and tumorigenicity [113, 114]. Pre-clinical studies have shown these cells to possess neurogenic [115] and myogenic potential [68, 116]. Also, they can migrate to the site of muscle degeneration; repopulate the satellite cell pool facilitating muscle regeneration [68, 116] and can survive in the injected muscles for long periods of time [83] promoting long term regeneration. These cells constitute a combination of cells including MSCs, hematopoietic cells, monocytes. Macrophages, stromal cells, very-small embryonic like stem cells, progenitor cells, hemangioblasts, endothelial progenitor cells and tissue-committed stem cells [117]. These cells are known to exert therapeutic benefits mainly through paracrine effects (**Figure 6**). They secrete a broad spectrum of cytokines and growth factors that exert anti-inflammation and immunosuppression, inhibition of apoptosis, homing of endogenous satellite cells, angiogenesis, and regulation of metabolic pathways [118, 119]. In MD, muscle fiber degeneration is followed by an invasion of inflammatory cells such as macrophages and T-lymphocytes [120]. The latter play

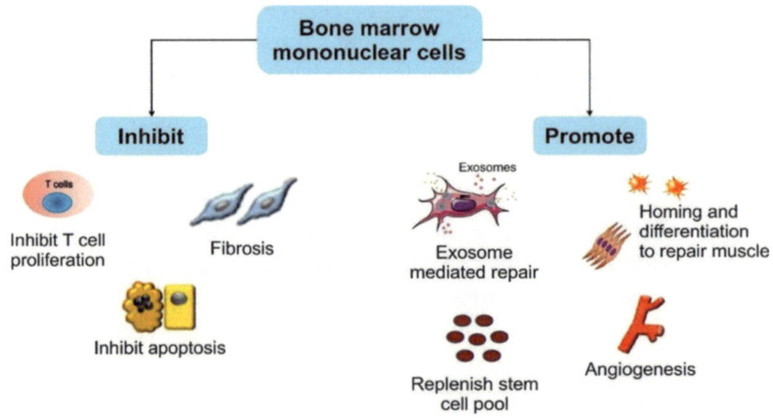

Figure 6.
Postulated mechanism of action of bone marrow mononuclear cells in MD.

a role in fibrosis which further hinders the ability of muscle fibers to regenerate. The anti-inflammatory effect of MSCs may provide protection from damage caused by T-lymphocytes [121]. Also, membrane derived vesicles, called as exosomes, arising from these cells may promote transcript transfer from the stem cells to the injured cells, causing injured cells to re-enter cell cycle further facilitating muscle repair [122, 123]. Though the ideal cell types for transplantation in MD continues to remain elusive, autologous bone marrow mononuclear cells are an attractive interim treatment solution with a potential to slow disease progression (**Figures** 7 and **8**).

6.2.2 Intrathecal and intramuscular delivery of cells

Occurrence of co-morbid intellectual disability and cognitive impairment in patients with DMD and BMD is suggestive of nervous system involvement in MDs [9, 10]. Dastur and Razzak found an overlap of pathological changes in muscle biopsy specimens of

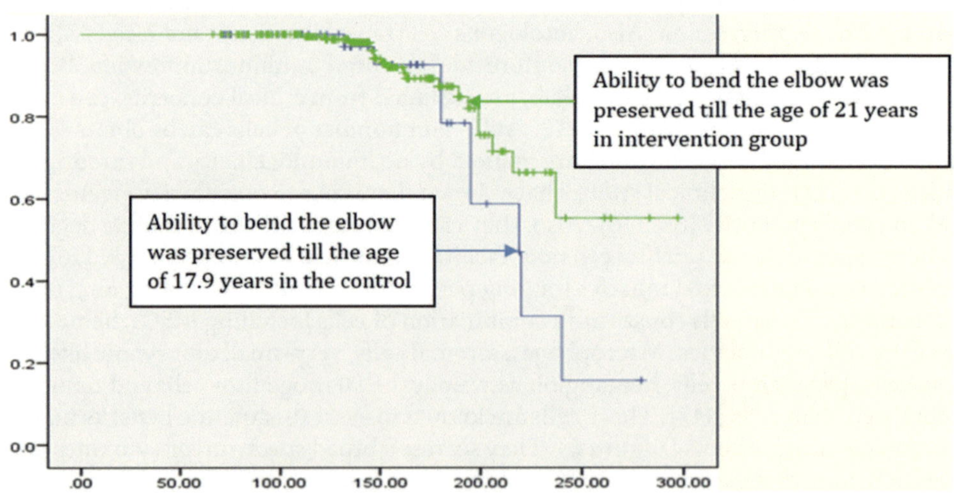

Figure 7.
Kaplan Meier graph showing comparison of the estimated time till loss of ability to lift the hand to mouth or deteriorate to the score of 5 on Brooke scale in intervention and control group.

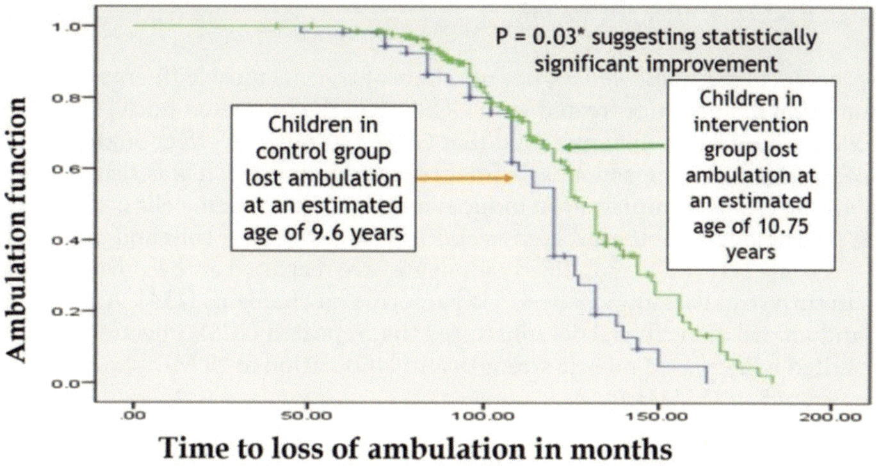

Figure 8.
Kaplan Meier graph showing comparison of the estimated time taken till loss of ambulation in intervention and control group.

patients with MD and patients with anterior horn cell disorders [124]. Histological study of the muscle biopsy specimens revealed small, atrophied muscle fibers in one fourth of the MD patients, suggesting a possible denervation and involvement of the neural systems in MD. These findings support intrathecal administration of stem cells and in our experience; it facilitates nerve repair and tightening of neuromuscular junction. Although intra-arterial and intravenous administration of stem cells is feasible because most of the skeletal muscles in the body are affected, only a small fraction of cells reaches the muscle tissue due to significant filtration of cells into the lungs, kidneys, and spleen [125, 126]. Moreover, the DGC is abundant at the neuromuscular junction and plays a role in neuromuscular homeostasis. Defects in DGC as in MD impair neuromuscular transmission and cause motor end plate abnormalities. Injecting the cells directly at motor points ensures repair of the nerve, muscle and myoneural synapse [30].

6.2.3 Combination of rehabilitation with cell therapy

Studies have investigated rehabilitation as a method to optimize cell therapy. Treadmill running following systemic transplantation of bone marrow derived MSCs in mouse models enhanced the contribution of donor cells in muscle fiber regeneration [127]. Endurance exercise results in an increase in blood levels of cytokines and an increase in bone marrow derived progenitor cells in humans. In response to exercise, there is an increase in secretion of vascular endothelial growth factor (VEGF) which is known to stimulate angiogenesis and satellite cell proliferation [128] and migration [129]. Intramuscular injection cannot be given in all the muscles and can only be given in selective muscles based on strength and accessibility. Widespread distribution and recruitment of circulatory stem cells is important which may be achieved through exercise. Long term, low-intensity, and low-load weight-bearing exercise programs may cause a shift in type II fibers to type I muscle fibers which are less susceptible to degeneration in MD [130]. Exercise increases expression of utrophin which is a homolog of dystrophin and can increase dystrophic muscle function [131]. Exercise also helps improve respiratory and cardiac function which is frequently affected in MD.

6.2.4 GCSF injection after cell therapy

A preclinical study showed higher numbers of normal muscle fibers and reduced inflammation in mdx mice treated with GCSF than the untreated mice [132]. A study in mdx mice model also demonstrated that GCSF has positive effect on the satellite cell proliferation and helps in muscle fiber regeneration [133]. It was also observed that periodic GCSF administration induces mobilization of stem cells including cells having proangiogenic potential such as endothelial progenitor cells and monocytes in MD patients [110]. The mobilized monocytes are recruited at the site of ischemia which in turn stimulate angiogenesis via paracrine mechanisms [134]. A prospective, non-randomized clinical trial demonstrated that repeated GCSF injections were safe and resulted in increased muscle strength and ambulation in 19 MD patients of age ranging from 5 to 15 [111].

6.2.5 Musculoskeletal magnetic resonance imaging

Skeletal muscle histopathology is a widely used tool in monitoring disease progression in MD cases; however, it is invasive, painful, gives limited information and might not be representative of the entire muscle [135]. In contrast, musculoskeletal MRI is a noninvasive technique and free of ionizing radiation. MRI-MSK provides information about all aspects of muscle structure and function and gives high resolution images of soft tissues and muscle fatty infiltrations [136]. MRI-MSK is sensitive to disease progression in MD and comparative MRI can serve as a biomarker for disease progression and to assess treatment efficacy [91–105, 137].

The efficacy of autologous bone marrow mononuclear cells in muscular dystrophy patients was studied and MRI-MSK was used as an outcome measure. After cell therapy patients showed increased muscle fibers in vastus medialis and lateralis (**Figure 9**), semitendinosus (**Figure 10**), tibialis (**Figure 11**), gastrocnemius (**Figures 12** and **13**), peroneus longus and brevis (**Figures 14** and **15**), triceps (**Figure 16**) and soleus (**Figure 17**) muscles.

6.3 Published results

A total of 15 studies (3 Cohort studies and 12 case reports) have been published that demonstrated the efficacy of autologous bone marrow mononuclear cell transplantation followed by rehabilitation in MD [91–105].

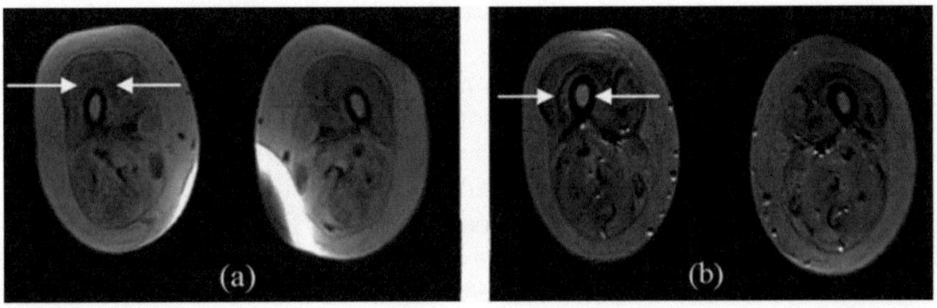

Figure 9.
(a) MRI scan of vastus medialis and lateralis muscles (arrows) pre-cell therapy. (b) MRI scan of vastus medialis and lateralis muscles (arrows) post- cell therapy showing muscle regeneration.

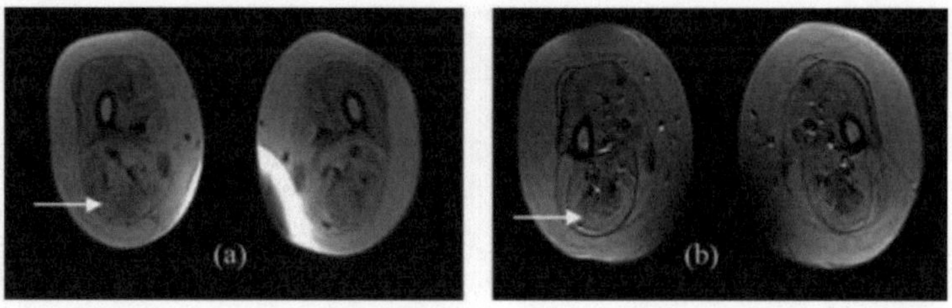

Figure 10.
(a) MRI scan of semitendinosus muscles (arrow) pre-cell therapy. (b) MRI scan of semitendinosus muscles (arrow) post-cell therapy showing muscle regeneration.

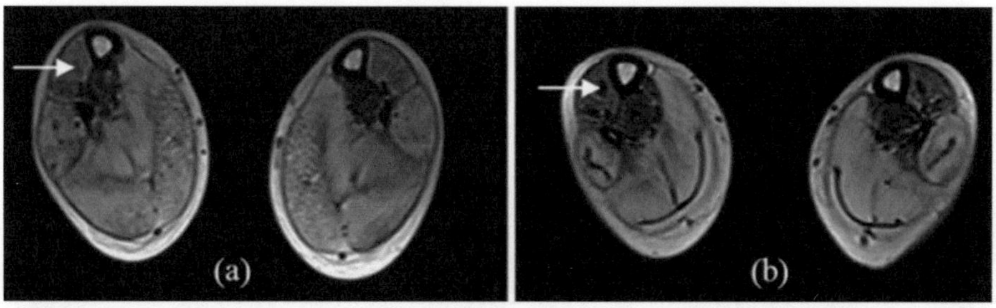

Figure 11.
(a) MRI scan of tibialis anterior (arrow) muscles pre-cell therapy. (b) MRI scan of tibialis anterior (arrow) muscles post-cell therapy showing muscle regeneration.

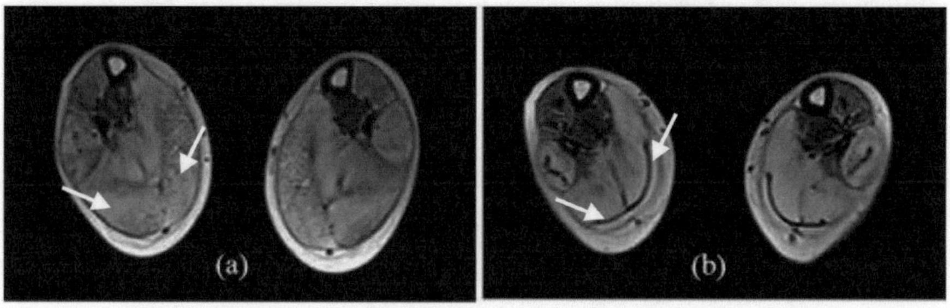

Figure 12.
(a) MRI scan of medial and lateral head of gastrocnemius muscle (arrow) muscles pre-cell therapy. (b) MRI scan of medial and lateral head of gastrocnemius muscle (arrow) muscles post-cell therapy showing muscle regeneration.

6.3.1 Results of published cohort studies

In 2012, a clinical study demonstrating the effect of bone marrow mononuclear cell transplantation in neurological and neuromuscular disorders in the pediatric population was published [97]. At a mean follow up of 15 ± 1 months post transplantation, 37 of the total38 patients with MD showed improvement in muscle strength (**Figure 18**). 73% showed improved trunk strength, 42% patients showed improvement in upper limb function and 71% patients showed improvement in lower limb function (**Figure 19**). Comparative musculoskeletal magnetic resonance imaging (MRI-MSK) done post intervention in two of the patients revealed decrease in fatty

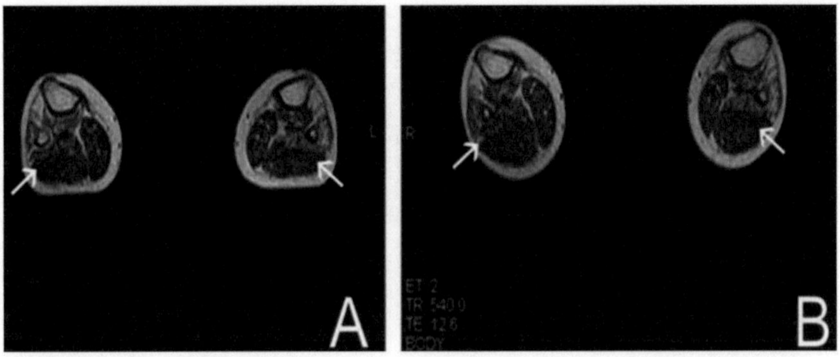

Figure 13.
(A) MRI scan of lateral head of gastrocnemius (arrow) pre-cell therapy. (B) MRI scan of lateral head of gastrocnemius (arrow) post-cell therapy showing muscle regeneration.

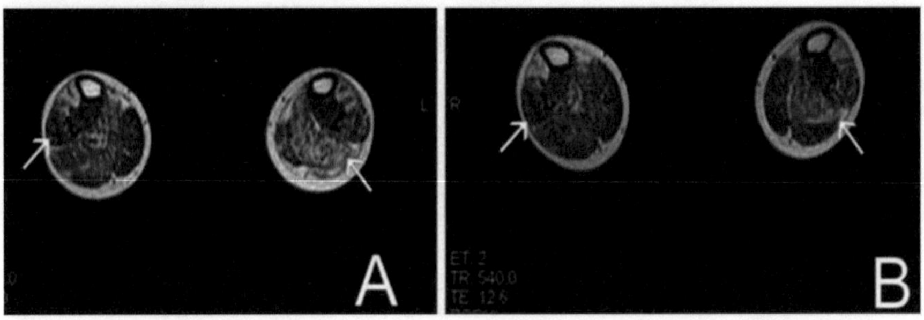

Figure 14.
(A) MRI scan showing peroneus longus and brevis (arrow) pre-cell therapy. (B) MRI scan showing peroneus longus and brevis (arrow) post cell therapy demonstrating muscle regeneration.

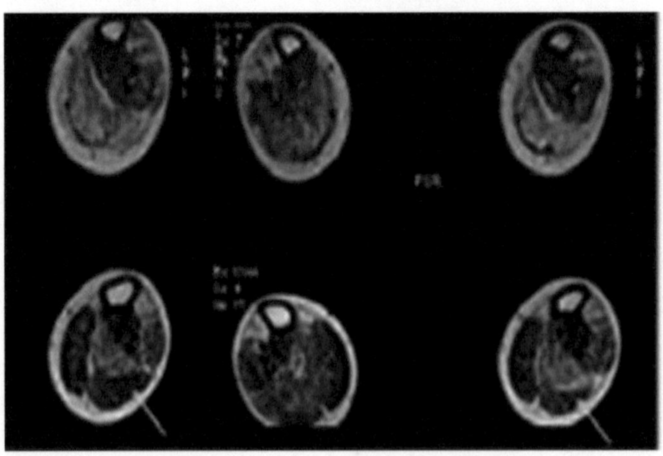

Figure 15.
Upper row. T1 weighted axial MRI images of peroneus longus and brevis, before cell therapy; lower row: T1 weighted axial MRI images of peroneus longus and brevis, 6 months post cell therapy showing increased isointense areas suggesting muscle regeneration.

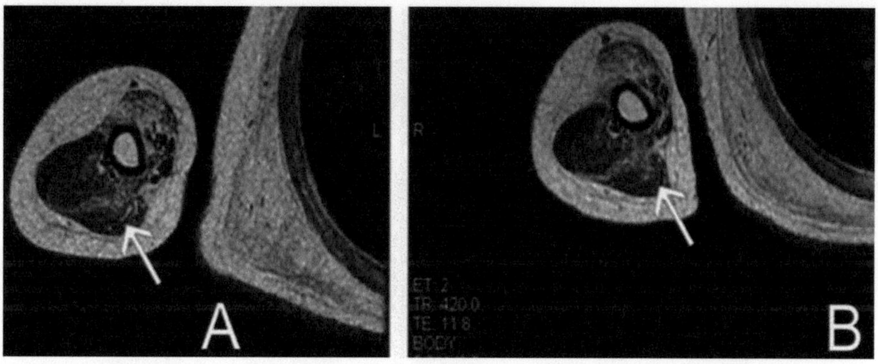

Figure 16.
(A) MRI scan of long, medial, and lateral head of triceps (arrow) pre-cell therapy. (B) MRI scan of long, medial, and lateral head of triceps (arrow) post-cell therapy showing muscle regeneration.

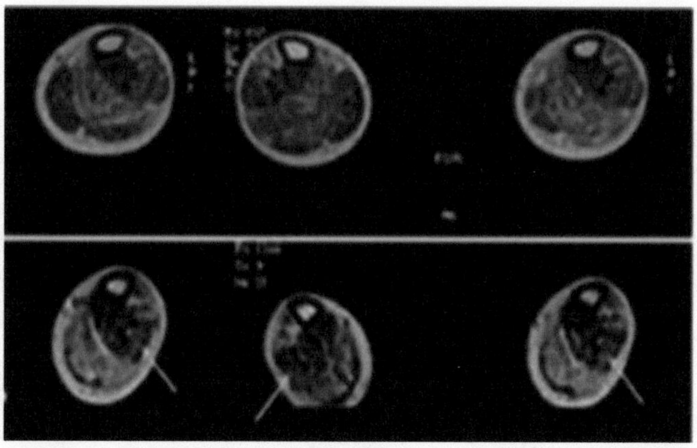

Figure 17.
Upper row: T1 weighted axial MRI images of gastrocnemius and soleus, before cell therapy. Lower row: T1 weighted axial MRI images gastrocnemius and soleus, 6 months after cell therapy showing increased isointense areas suggesting muscle regeneration.

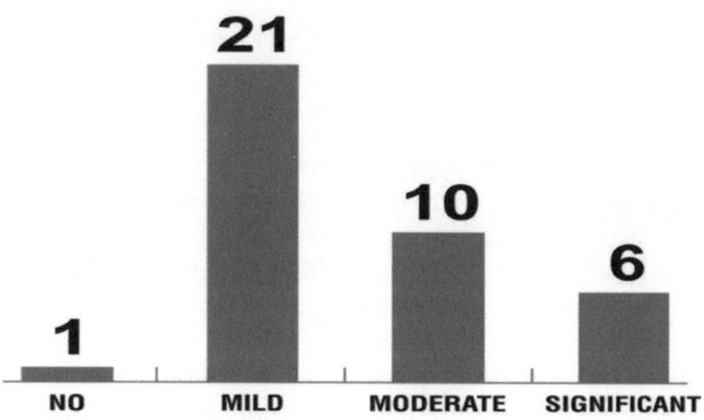

Figure 18.
Graph showing improvement in patients with MD post cell therapy.

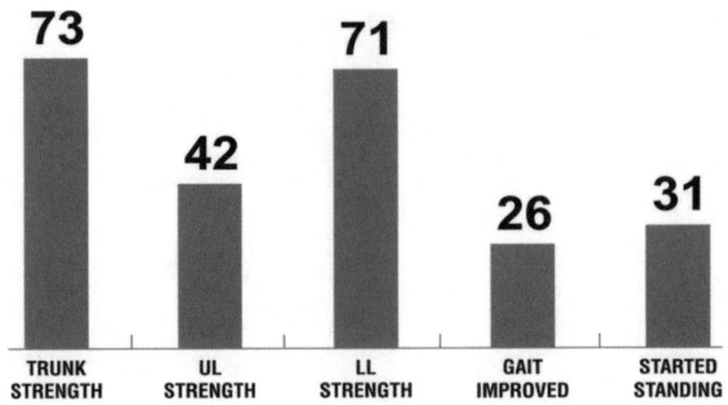

Figure 19.
Graph representing symptom-wise improvements in MD patients post cell therapy.

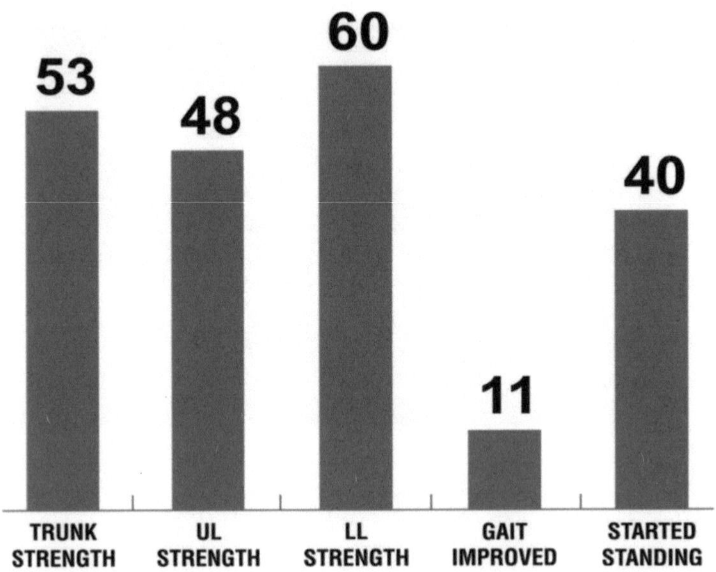

Figure 20.
Graph showing symptom wise improvements in muscular dystrophy patients after stem cell therapy. Number of patients showing improvements with respect to trunk strength, upper limb (UL) strength, lower limb (LL) strength, gait, and standing are shown.

infiltration with minimal muscle regeneration seen mostly in the muscles that had received cells (**Figures 9–12**). Improved muscle electrical activity was noted in 3 patients on comparative EMG done post intervention.

In 2013 an open label study that included 150 patients with MD was published [91]. On a mean follow up of 12 ± 1 months, 86.67% cases showed strength improvement with 53% patients showed improvement in trunk strength and 60% patients improving in lower limb strength (**Figure 20**). Improvements were seen on EMG in 9 cases and 6 cases showed improvement on MRI-MSK (**Figures 13, 14** and **16**).

A longitudinal study of 65 LGMD patients was published in 2015 [98]. Depending on the number of transplants, the patients were divided into 3 groups. Group 1 included patients that underwent single transplantation, group 2 included patients that underwent 2 transplantations and group 3 included patients that underwent 3 transplantations. 97% of patients displayed improved function on FIM scale in group 1. Statistically significant strength improvements were noted 6 months post transplantation. In group 2, 96% of the patients displayed improved function on FIM scale. Statistically significant strength improvements were noted 6 months post intervention. In group 3, of the 4 patients, 1 patient deteriorated in FIM score, 2 patients improved and in 1 patient, the FIM score was maintained. Most patients had maintained muscle strength. The patient who showed deterioration in FIM score also showed deterioration in muscle strength. This patient had come for the cell therapy at an advanced stage of the disease, where the muscle strength was minimal, and he was completely dependent for all his activities of daily living.

6.3.2 Results of published case reports

Though at a variable rate, progressive skeletal muscle weakness is consistent with all the MD variants. The improvements after cellular therapy was measured on various outcome measures which are as follows-

a. 6-minute walk test

Improvement was seen in the case of BMD in the 6-minute walk test. Maintenance and even improvement of function on the 6-minute walk test, over a follow up period of 1 year, was reported in two individual cases of DMD post intervention [94, 101]. Improvement also observed in a case of LGMD patient (94a). Considering the progressive nature of the disease, the natural decline shown by MD ambulant patients is 22.7 meters in the first year and 64.7 meters in the second year [138] which is slowed down because of cellular therapy.

b. North star ambulatory Assessment (NSAA)

Improvement was observed in DMD and BMD patients in North star ambulatory Assessment scale [92, 101, 102]. In a published case report, a DMD patient of 10 years of age showed a maintained score on NSAA after 13 months of follow up [93] which shows positive effects of cellular therapy as there is continuous decrease in the scores of NSAA in DMD patients after 7 years of age [138].

c. Brooke and Vignos Scales

The improvements are also observed in Brooke and Vignos scales that measure the strength of upper and lower extremity respectively. The improvement in ambulation and gait contributed toward a positive shift on Brooke and Vignos Scales in MD patients [91, 97]. Improved scores also observed in a case of DMD [103]. The scores are maintained on two cases of BMD which shows the efficacy of SCT considering the progressive nature of the disease.

d. Functional Independence Measure

The improved functional independence measure (FIM) score is observed after cellular therapy in most of the BMD, DMD and LGMD patients and is evident by improved quality of life in those patients [91, 93, 97–99, 102, 103]. In two BMD and one LGMD patient the score was maintained demonstrating the halted disease progression [92, 95, 100].

e. Manual muscle Testing (MMT)

The efficacy of cellular therapy was also assessed by MMT score. There are improvements observed in MMT grading which is attributed to improved muscle strength in many DMD, BMD and LGMD patients [91, 95, 96, 98–104]. In a DMD patient, though the grading did not change but the control and quality of movement had improved, grip strength and pinch strength also showed minimal changes on both sides [100]. This indicates alteration in the disease progression, as the natural course of the disease shows reduction of muscular strength by 0.3 MMT units/year and 3.9% reduction in muscle strength every year [103].

f. MRI-MSK

Comparative MRI-MSK was done to study the efficacy of cellular therapy. The comparative MRI-MSK findings showed no increase in the fatty infiltration in BMD, DMD and LGMD patients [96, 99, 101–103, 105]. BMD is associated with progressive increase in fatty infiltration of muscle tissue and the comparison of MRI scans of children with DMD also suggests a 5% increase of fatty infiltration every year [139]. Thus, no significant increase in the fatty infiltration shows the effectiveness of cellular therapy in halting the disease progression. Decrease in fatty infiltration was reported in a case of BMD in bilateral peroneus longus and brevis muscle fibers (**Figures 14** and **15**) 6 months post intervention [100].

g. Electromyography (EMG)

Comparative EMG-NCV (EMG-nerve conduction velocity) showed no increase in the dystrophic changes of the muscles, suggesting maintained muscle integrity suggesting altered disease progression [99]. In a DMD patient, EMG studies showed improvement in the recruitment of the vastus medialis muscle, which is a key muscle in patellar stability and knee stability while walking which was functionally reflected as the ability to stand and walk independently, maintained over 3 years [103]. A decrease in extramyocellular lipid (EMCL) resonance peak was seen in a case of LGMD [96]. The EMCL quantifies fat content in a diseased muscle. Improvement in electrical activity of muscle on EMG also observed in 9 patients post cellular therapy [91].

6.3.3 Adverse events

All these preliminary studies demonstrated safety of cell therapy using intrathecal and intramuscular transplantation of autologous bone marrow mononuclear cells. These studies encountered no procedure related major complications. 3 studies reported minor adverse events which included headache, nausea, vomiting, backache, and pain at injection site [91, 97, 98]. These were self-limiting and resolved within a week.

7. Unpublished results

7.1 DMD

A total of 296 patients with DMD underwent autologous transplantation of bone marrow mononuclear cells by intrathecal and intramuscular routes followed

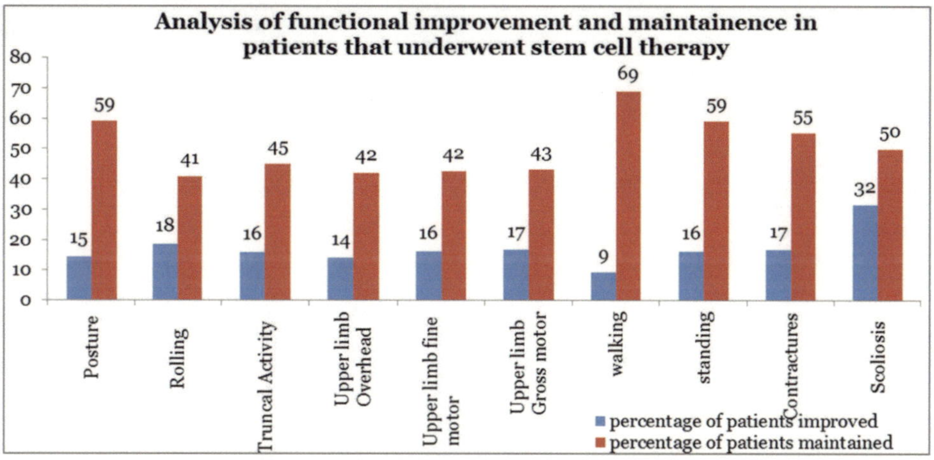

Figure 21.
Graph showing percentage analysis of symptoms in DMD patients post cell therapy.

by rehabilitation. There were no major side effects. 5.4% patients experienced minor procedural adverse events which included spinal headache, fever, nausea and vomiting, pain at aspiration site, backache, neck pain, pain in lower limbs and loose motions. These were self-limiting and resolved within a week with medications. 55 patients that only received standard treatment for DMD formed the control group.

On a follow-up period ranging from 6 months to 78 months (median 18 months), 76% patients showed symptomatic and functional maintenance and/or improvements (**Figure 21**). The natural course of DMD being progressive, symptomatic, or functional maintenance or improvement were considered together.

7.1.1 Effect of cell therapy on muscle strength

Difference between muscle strength on MMT in individual muscle groups at the first and last assessment at mean follow up duration of 12.2 ± 8.6 months was analyzed using Wilcoxon signed rank test. Except for hip extensors, knee extensors and shoulder flexors, all muscle groups had maintained muscle strength. Also, there was a statistically significant increase in muscle strength post intervention in the wrist flexors. Overall muscle strength (%MRC) was calculated for each patient. Difference between %MRC at the first and last assessment was analyzed using the Wilcoxon signed rank test (**Table 1**). We found a statistically insignificant decline in %MRC of 1.04% in patients aged 5–13 years, over mean follow up of 12.2 ± 8.6 months. This was lower than the annual decline of 3.9% in natural controls [140]. There was a statistically insignificant increase of 0.92% in %MRC in patients aged 14 years or more. A 2% annual decline in %MRC in this age group has been reported in previous literature [141].

7.1.2 Comparison of functional decline between treatment and control group

On comparing the predicted age at which patients could not lift their hand to the mouth and lost their ability to self-feed (Brooke score declining to 5) using Kaplan-Meier analysis, patients that received cell therapy reached score 5 at age 21 years while patients that did not receive cell therapy reached the score at age 18 years (**Figure 7**

Variables	MMT score		% MRC		Significance
	Before intervention	After intervention	Before intervention	After intervention	
Mean Score (5–13 years age group)	9.15	8.98	57.19%	56.15%	p = 0.1031
Mean Score (>14 years age group)	5.87	6.01	36.67%	37.59%	p = 0.0750

Table 1.
Results of analysis of overall manual strength (%MRC) before and after intervention in the age group 5–13 years and > 14 years at a mean follow up of 12 months (p < 0.05 was considered statistically significant).

	Control Group(months)	Intervention Group (months)	Statistical significance
Total no. of patients	55	139	—
Estimated time to loss of ambulation in months	117	130	0.006*
Estimated time to reach score of 5 on Brooke scale	216	252	0.150
Estimated time of survival	260	297	0.173

Table 2.
*Results of Kaplan Meier analysis in intervention and control group (*indicates statistically significant difference between the groups).*

and **Table 2**). This difference of 36 months was clinically meaningful however not statistically significant ($p = 0.150$).

Comparing the predicted age to loss of ambulation using Kaplan-Meier analysis, the predicted time to loss of ambulation was 130 months in the cell therapy group and 117 months in the control group (**Figure 8** and **Table 2**). There was a statistically significant ($p < 0.05$) increase in time to loss of ambulation by 13 months in the cell therapy group.

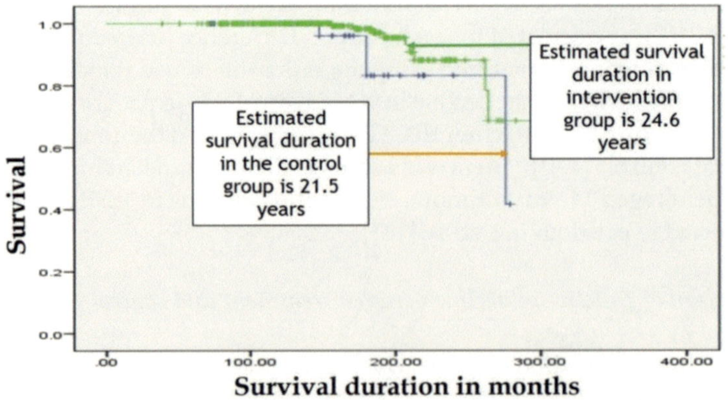

Figure 22.
Kaplan Meier graph showing comparison of estimated survival duration of the intervention and control group.

On comparing the survival duration using Kaplan-Meier analysis, the estimated survival duration of patients that received cell therapy was 297 months, while that of the control group was 260 months (**Figure 22**). Though statistically insignificant ($p = 0.173$), there was an increase in estimated survival duration by 37 months in the cell therapy group.

8. Summary of effects of SCT in MD

MD is considered as stem cell disease as symptoms are visible only after depletion of the stem cell pool. Therefore, replenishment of the stem cell pool is necessary to ameliorate the symptoms. This can be achieved by stem cell therapy which is found to be a safe and effective treatment strategy for MD. SCT delays the progression of the disease, improves functionality and quality of life of MD patients. SCT in combination with rehabilitation and GCSF administration gives better results. The effects of SCT may be further enhanced by other integrative therapies such as hyperbaric oxygen therapy (HBOT), ozone therapy and deep tissue mobilization (DTM). These therapies may help to fasten the process of regeneration and repair because of their therapeutic effects.

9. Integrative therapies in MD

9.1 Hyperbaric oxygen therapy (HBOT)

The pathophysiology of MD patients includes vascular dysfunction, altered angiogenesis, hypoxia, inflammation, and ischemia [142]. Studies have shown that HBOT enhances healing of wounds, ischemia, and inflammations [143]. It also reduces hypoxia and increases angiogenesis by inducing secretion of VEGF (Vascular endothelial growth factor) and bFGF (basic fibroblast growth factor) [144]. Thereby, HBOT is a promising therapy to ameliorate the condition of MD individuals. A study revealed that HBOT promotes muscle regeneration and satellite cell proliferation in mouse skeletal muscles injury models [145]. Thom et al. demonstrated that exposure to HBOT rapidly mobilizes stem progenitor cells in humans and mice [146]. Thus, HBOT in combination with stem cell therapy can show better therapeutic effects. HBOT stimulates neurogenesis and synaptogenesis, thereby improving motor functions and cognitive functions [147]. Leitman et al. demonstrated that HBOT also improves myocardial functions which are profoundly affected in MD patients [148].

9.2 Ozone therapy

Ozone therapy enhances tissue oxygenation and improves cellular metabolism. It also reduces oxidative stress and inflammation [149]. Preclinical study has shown that dystrophin deficient mdx mice have increased reactive oxygen species (ROS) levels in their heart which play a critical role in the development of dilated cardiomyopathy and inflammation of heart [150]. Also, Myofiber necrosis in MD patients is closely associated with increased inflammation and ROS levels [151]. The anti-inflammatory and antioxidant properties of ozone therapy may help in limiting disease progression by reducing oxidative stress and inflammation in MD patients. Ozone therapy also helps in mobilization of stem cells and homing of stem cells toward injured/ischemic sites, thus, aid in tissue repair [152]. This evidence suggests that stem cell therapy in combination with ozone therapy may show better therapeutic efficacy in MD patients.

9.3 Deep tissue mobilization (DTM)

Soft tissue mobilization helps in removing scars and soft tissue regeneration after injury [153]. Massage therapy reduces inflammation and promotes angiogenesis in the injured tissues after muscle damage [154]. In 20 DMD patients, calf massage showed increase in calf and hamstring muscle length and reduction in calf muscle stiffness [155]. Thereby, DTM is a beneficial option in cases of MD as they have increased inflammation [151]. An increased level of profibrotic factor TGFβ1 is observed in muscles of DMD patients [156] which is reduced by brief stretching of tissue beyond the habitual range [157]. A preclinical study demonstrated that massage therapy in 32 rats have increased satellite cell number in their gastrocnemius muscle [158]. This finding suggests that DTM along with stem cell therapy is a beneficial option for the treatment of MD.

10. Future directions and conclusion

Clearly, the initiation of disease pathology is due to genetic defect, but progression is due to satellite cell exhaustion and loss of regenerative capacity of satellite cells. Replenishing satellite cell pool and enhancing regenerative capacity of muscle fibers is essential for any treatment to be effective. Cell therapy represents a potential treatment strategy for MD. Goals that need to be fulfilled include delivery of normal protein to affected muscle fibers, effective fusion of donor cells to affected muscle fibers, delivery of large numbers of stem cells, repopulating of the resident stem cell pool, long term survival of stem cells to facilitate long term muscle repair and homeostasis. All these goals may not be met using one cell type and may require a combination of cell therapies. Future studies could explore systemic delivery of cells along with transplantation of different types of autologous/allogeneic cells in larger numbers intramuscularly and/or with intrathecal administration. Studies could also combine the genetic therapies with stem cell replacement to identify the most effective cure for DMD. Larger randomized studies to determine the ideal cell combination, route of delivery and cell dosage are recommended. Studies can also explore the effects of cellular therapy in combination with integrative therapies such as HBOT, ozone therapy and DTM.

Author details

Alok Sharma, Hemangi Sane, Nandini Gokulchandran, Amruta Paranjape*, Zubiya Shaikh, Arjun KM and Prerna Badhe
Neurogen Brain and Spine Institute, Navi Mumbai, India

*Address all correspondence to: amrutap.neurogen@gmail.com

IntechOpen

© 2023 The Author(s). Licensee IntechOpen. This chapter is distributed under the terms of the Creative Commons Attribution License (http://creativecommons.org/licenses/by/3.0), which permits unrestricted use, distribution, and reproduction in any medium, provided the original work is properly cited.

References

[1] Gardner-Medwin D. Clinical features and classification of the muscular dystrophies. British Medical Bulletin. 1980;**36**(2):109-116

[2] Cohn RD, Campbell KP. Molecular basis of muscular dystrophies. Muscle & Nerve. 2000;**23**(10):1456-1471

[3] Bornemann A, Anderson LVB. Diagnostic protein expression in human muscle biopsies. Brain Pathology. 2000;**10**(2):193-214

[4] Salari N, Fatahi B, Valipour E, Kazeminia M, Fatahian R, Kiaei A, et al. Global prevalence of Duchenne and Becker muscular dystrophy: A systematic review and meta-analysis. Journal of Orthopaedic Surgery and Research. 2022;**17**(1):96

[5] Mercuri E, Muntoni F. Muscular d ystrophies. The Lancet. 2013;**381**(9869): 845-860

[6] Coral-Vazquez R, Cohn RD, Moore SA, Hill JA, Weiss RM, Davisson RL, et al. Disruption of the Sarcoglycan–Sarcospan complex in vascular smooth muscle: A novel mechanism for cardiomyopathy and muscular dystrophy. Cell. 1999;**98**(4):465-474

[7] Moore SA, Saito F, Chen J, Michele DE, Henry MD, Messing A, et al. Deletion of brain dystroglycan recapitulates aspects of congenital muscular dystrophy. Nature. 2002;**418**(6896):422-425

[8] Michele DE, Barresi R, Kanagawa M, Saito F, Cohn RD, Satz JS, et al. Post-translational disruption of dystroglycan–ligand interactions in congenital muscular dystrophies. Nature. 2002;**418**(6896):417-421

[9] Pane M, Lombardo ME, Alfieri P, D'Amico A, Bianco F, Vasco G, et al. Attention deficit hyperactivity disorder and cognitive function in Duchenne muscular dystrophy: Phenotype-genotype correlation. The Journal of Pediatrics. 2012;**161**(4):705-9.e1

[10] Cyrulnik SE, Fee RJ, Batchelder A, Kiefel J, Goldstein E, Hinton VJ. Cognitive and adaptive deficits in young children with Duchenne muscular dystrophy (DMD). Journal of International Neuropsychology Society. 2008;**14**(5):853-861

[11] Engel AG, Franzini-Armstrong C, editors. Myology: Basic and Clinical. 2nd ed. New York: McGraw-Hill; 1994. p. 1937

[12] Campbell KP. Three muscular dystrophies: Loss of cytoskeleton-extracellular matrix linkage. Cell. 1995;**80**(5):675-679

[13] Petrof BJ, Shrager JB, Stedman HH, Kelly AM, Sweeney HL. Dystrophin protects the sarcolemma from stresses developed during muscle contraction. Proceedings of the National Academy of Sciences USA. 1993;**90**(8):3710-3714

[14] Weller B, Karpati G, Carpenter S. Dystrophin-deficient mdx muscle fibers are preferentially vulnerable to necrosis induced by experimental lengthening contractions. Journal of the Neurological Sciences. 1990;**100**(1-2):9-13

[15] Spence HJ, Chen Y-J, Winder SJ. Muscular dystrophies, the cytoskeleton and cell adhesion. BioEssays. 2002;**24**(6):542-552

[16] Blake DJ, Weir A, Newey SE, Davies KE. Function and genetics of dystrophin and dystrophin-related

proteins in muscle. Physiological Reviews. 2002;**82**(2):291-329

[17] Górecki DC. Prospects and problems of gene therapy: An update. Expert Opinion on Emerging Drugs. 2001;**6**(2):187-198

[18] Matsuo M. Antisense oligonucleotide-mediated exon-skipping therapies: Precision medicine spreading from duchenne muscular dystrophy. JMA Journal. 2021;**4**(3):232-240

[19] Blau HM, Webster C, Pavlath GK. Defective myoblasts identified in Duchenne muscular dystrophy. PNAS. 1983;**80**(15):4856-4860

[20] Renault V, Piron-Hamelin G, Forestier C, DiDonna S, Decary S, Hentati F, et al. Skeletal muscle regeneration and the mitotic clock. Experimental Gerontology. 2000;**35**(6): 711-719

[21] Sacco A, Mourkioti F, Tran R, Choi J, Llewellyn M, Kraft P, et al. Short telomeres and stem cell exhaustion model Duchenne muscular dystrophy in mdx/mTR mice. Cell. 2010;**143**(7):1059-1071

[22] McDouall RM, Dunn MJ, Dubowitz V. Nature of the mononuclear infiltrate and the mechanism of muscle damage in juvenile dermatomyositis and Duchenne muscular dystrophy. Journal of the Neurological Sciences. 1990;**99**(2-3):199-217

[23] Morrison J, Palmer DB, Cobbold S, Partridge T, Bou-Gharios G. Effects of T-lymphocyte depletion on muscle fibrosis in the mdx mouse. The American Journal of Pathology. 2005;**166**(6):1701-1710

[24] Morrison J, Lu QL, Pastoret C, Partridge T, Bou-Gharios G. T-cell-dependent fibrosis in the mdx dystrophic mouse. Laboratory Investigation. 2000;**80**(6):881-891

[25] Mann CJ, Perdiguero E, Kharraz Y, Aguilar S, Pessina P, Serrano AL, et al. Aberrant repair and fibrosis development in skeletal muscle. Skeletal Muscle. 2011;**1**(1):21

[26] Nowak KJ, Davies KE. Duchenne muscular dystrophy and dystrophin: Pathogenesis and opportunities for treatment. EMBO Reports. 2004;**5**(9):872-876

[27] Tidball JG, Wehling-Henricks M. Damage and inflammation in muscular dystrophy: Potential implications and relationships with autoimmune myositis. Current Opinion in Rheumatology. 2005;**17**(6):707-713

[28] Tews DS. Apoptosis and muscle fibre loss in neuromuscular disorders. Neuromuscular Disorders. 2002;**12**(7-8):613-622

[29] Haenggi T, Fritschy JM. Role of dystrophin and utrophin for assembly and function of the dystrophin glycoprotein complex in non-muscle tissue. Cellular and Molecular Life Sciences. 2006;**63**:1614-1631

[30] Pilgram GS, Potikanond S, Baines RA, Fradkin LG, Noordermeer JN. The roles of the dystrophin-associated glycoprotein complex at the synapse. Molecular Neurobiology. 2010;**41**(1):1-21

[31] Liesveld JL, Sharma N, Aljitawi OS. Stem cell homing: From physiology to therapeutics. Stem Cells. 2020;**38**:1241-1253

[32] Vieira NM, Brandalise V, Zucconi E, Jazedje T, Secco M, Nunes VA, et al. Human multipotent adipose-derived stem cells restore dystrophin expression of Duchenne skeletal-muscle

cells in vitro. Biology of the Cell. 2008;**100**(4):231-241

[33] Baraniak PR, McDevitt TC. Stem cell paracrine actions and tissue regeneration. Regenerative Medicine. 2010;**5**(1):121-143

[34] Negroni E, Gidaro T, Bigot A, Butler-Browne GS, Mouly V, Trollet C. Invited review: Stem cells and muscle diseases: Advances in cell therapy strategies. Neuropathology and Applied Neurobiology. 2015;**41**(3):270-287

[35] Young HE, Black AC. Adult stem cells. The Anatomical Record Part A: Discoveries in Molecular, Cellular, and Evolutionary Biology. 2004;**276A**(1):75-102

[36] Zakrzewski W, Dobrzyński M, Szymonowicz M, Rybak Z. Stem cells: Past, present, and future. Stem Cell Research & Therapy. 2019;**10**(1):1-22

[37] Takahashi K, Yamanaka S. Induction of pluripotent stem cells from mouse embryonic and adult fibroblast cultures by defined factors. Cell. 2006;**126**(4):663-676

[38] Awaya T, Kato T, Mizuno Y, Chang H, Niwa A, Umeda K, et al. Selective development of myogenic mesenchymal cells from human embryonic and induced pluripotent stem cells. PLoS One. 2012;**7**(12):e51638

[39] Goudenege S, Lebel C, Huot NB, Dufour C, Fujii I, Gekas J, et al. Myoblasts derived from normal hESCs and dystrophic hiPSCs efficiently fuse with existing muscle fibers following transplantation. Molecular Therapy. 2012;**20**(11):2153-2167

[40] Darabi R, Arpke RW, Irion S, Dimos JT, Grskovic M, Kyba M, et al. Human ES- and iPS-derived myogenic progenitors restore dystrophin and improve contractility upon transplantation in dystrophic mice. Cell Stem Cell. 2012;**10**(5):610-619

[41] Zammit PS, Partridge TA, Yablonka-Reuveni Z. The skeletal muscle satellite cell: The stem cell that came in from the cold. Journal of Histochemistry Cytochemistry. 2006;**54**(11):1177-1191

[42] Allen RE, Dodson MV, Luiten LS, Boxhorn LK. A serum-free medium that supports the growth of cultured skeletal muscle satellite cells. In Vitro Cellular & Developmental Biology. 1985;**21**(11):636-640

[43] Bischoff R. Proliferation of muscle satellite cells on intact myofibers in culture. Developmental Biology. 1986;**115**(1):129-139

[44] Morgan JE, Watt DJ, Sloper JC, Partridge TA. Partial correction of an inherited biochemical defect of skeletal muscle by grafts of normal muscle precursor cells. Journal of the Neurological Sciences. 1988;**86**(2):137-147

[45] Partridge TA, Morgan JE, Coulton GR, Hoffman EP, Kunkel LM. Conversion of mdx myofibres from dystrophin-negative to -positive by injection of normal myoblasts. Nature. 1989;**337**(6203):176-179

[46] Morgan JE, Pagel CN, Sherrratt T, Partridge TA. Long-term persistence and migration of myogenic cells injected into pre-irradiated muscles of mdx mice. Journal of the Neurological Sciences. 1993;**115**(2):191-200

[47] Ikezawa M, Cao B, Qu Z, Peng H, Xiao X, Pruchnic R, et al. Dystrophin delivery in dystrophin-deficient DMDmdx skeletal muscle by isogenic muscle-derived stem cell

transplantation. Human Gene Therapy. 2003;**14**(16):1535-1546

[48] Qu-Petersen Z, Deasy B, Jankowski R, Ikezawa M, Cummins J, Pruchnic R, et al. Identification of a novel population of muscle stem cells in mice: Potential for muscle regeneration. The Journal of Cell Biology. 2002;**157**(5):851-864

[49] Huard J, Cao B, Qu-Petersen Z. Muscle-derived stem cells: Potential for muscle regeneration. Birth Defects Research Part C: Embryo Today: Reviews. 2003;**69**(3):230-237

[50] Minasi MG, Riminucci M, Angelis LD, Borello U, Berarducci B, Innocenzi A, et al. The meso-angioblast: A multipotent, self-renewing cell that originates from the dorsal aorta and differentiates into most mesodermal tissues. Development. 2002;**129**(11):2773-2783

[51] Cossu G, Bianco P. Mesoangioblasts — vascular progenitors for extravascular mesodermal tissues. Current Opinion in Genetics & Development. 2003;**13**(5):537-542

[52] Galvez BG, Sampaolesi M, Brunelli S, Covarello D, Gavina M, Rossi B, et al. Complete repair of dystrophic skeletal muscle by mesoangioblasts with enhanced migration ability. The Journal of Cell Biology. 2006;**174**(2):231-243

[53] Asakura A, Seale P, Girgis-Gabardo A, Rudnicki MA. Myogenic specification of side population cells in skeletal muscle. The Journal of Cell Biology. 2002;**159**(1):123-134

[54] Rouger K, Larcher T, Dubreil L, Deschamps J-Y, Le Guiner C, Jouvion G, et al. Systemic delivery of allogenic muscle stem cells induces long-term muscle repair and clinical efficacy in Duchenne muscular dystrophy dogs. The American Journal of Pathology. 2011;**179**(5):2501-2518

[55] Tedesco FS, Dellavalle A, Diaz-Manera J, Messina G, Cossu G. Repairing skeletal muscle: Regenerative potential of skeletal muscle stem cells. The Journal of Clinical Investigation. 2010;**120**(1):11-19

[56] Sampaolesi M, Torrente Y, Innocenzi A, Tonlorenzi R, D'Antona G, Pellegrino MA, et al. Cell therapy of α-Sarcoglycan null dystrophic mice through intra-arterial delivery of Mesoangioblasts. Science. 2003;**301**(5632):487-492

[57] Guttinger M, Tafi E, Battaglia M, Coletta M, Cossu G. Allogeneic mesoangioblasts give rise to alpha-sarcoglycan expressing fibers when transplanted into dystrophic mice. Experimental Cell Research. 2006;**312**(19):3872-3879

[58] Sampaolesi M, Blot S, D'Antona G, Granger N, Tonlorenzi R, Innocenzi A, et al. Mesoangioblast stem cells ameliorate muscle function in dystrophic dogs. Nature. 2006;**444**(7119):574-579

[59] Dellavalle A, Sampaolesi M, Tonlorenzi R, Tagliafico E, Sacchetti B, Perani L, et al. Pericytes of human skeletal muscle are myogenic precursors distinct from satellite cells. Nature Cell Biology. 2007;**9**(3):255-267

[60] Boldrin L, Morgan JE. Activating muscle stem cells: Therapeutic potential in muscle diseases. Current Opinion in Neurology. 2007;**20**(5):577

[61] Torrente Y, Belicchi M, Sampaolesi M, Pisati F, Meregalli M, D'Antona G, et al. Human circulating AC133(+) stem cells restore dystrophin expression and ameliorate function

in dystrophic skeletal muscle. The Journal of Clinical Investigation. 2004;**114**(2):182-195

[62] Péault B, Rudnicki M, Torrente Y, Cossu G, Tremblay JP, Partridge T, et al. Stem and progenitor cells in skeletal muscle development, maintenance, and therapy. Molecular Therapy. 2007;**15**(5):867-877

[63] Benchaouir R, Meregalli M, Farini A, D'Antona G, Belicchi M, Goyenvalle A, et al. Restoration of human dystrophin following transplantation of exon-skipping-engineered DMD patient stem cells into dystrophic mice. Cell Stem Cell. 2007;**1**(6):646-657

[64] Laumonier T, Bermont F, Hoffmeyer P, Kindler V, Menetrey J. Human myogenic reserve cells are quiescent stem cells that contribute to muscle regeneration after intramuscular transplantation in immunodeficient mice. Scientific Reports. 2017;**7**(1):1-2

[65] Bongso A, Lee EH. Stem cells: From Bench to Bed Side. In: Bongso A, Lee EH, editors. World Scientific. Singapore; 2005. pp. 1-13. [cited 2018 Nov 12]. Available From: https://www.worldscientific.com/doi/abs/10.1142/9789812569370_0001

[66] Ferrari G, Cusella G, Angelis D, Coletta M, Paolucci E, Stornaiuolo A, et al. Muscle regeneration by bone marrow-derived myogenic progenitors. Science. 1998;**279**(5356):1528-1530

[67] Gussoni E, Soneoka Y, Strickland CD, Buzney EA, Khan MK, Flint AF, et al. Dystrophin expression in the mdx mouse restored by stem cell transplantation. Nature. 1999;**401**(6751):390

[68] Maeda Y, Yonemochi Y, Nakajyo Y, Hidaka H, Ikeda T, Ando Y. CXCL12 and osteopontin from bone marrow-derived mesenchymal stromal cells improve muscle regeneration. Scientific Reports. 2017;**7**(1):1-1

[69] Park SE, Jeong JB, Oh SJ, Kim SJ, Kim H, Choi A, et al. Wharton's jelly-derived mesenchymal stem cells reduce fibrosis in a mouse model of Duchenne muscular dystrophy by upregulating microRNA 499. Biomedicine. 2021;**9**(9):1089

[70] Law P, Bertorini T, Goodwin T, Chen M, Fang Q, Li H-J, et al. Dystrophin production induced by myoblast transfer therapy in Duchenne muscular dystrophy. The Lancet. 1990;**336**(8707):114-115

[71] Neumeyer AM, Cross D, McKenna-Yasek D, Zawadzka A, Hoffman EP, Pegoraro E, et al. Pilot study of myoblast transfer in the treatment of Becker muscular dystrophy. Neurology. 1998;**51**(2):589

[72] Law PK, Goodwin TG, Fang Q, Chen M, Li H-J, Florendo JA, et al. Myoblast transfer therapy for Duchenne muscular dystrophy. Pediatrics International. 1991;**33**(2):206-215

[73] Karpati G, Ajdukovic D, Arnold D, Gledhill RB, Guttmann R, Holland P, et al. Myoblast transfer in duchenne muscular dystrophy. Annals of Neurology. 1993;**34**(1):8-17

[74] Morandi L, Bernasconi P, Gebbia M, Mora M, Crosti F, Mantegazza R, et al. Lack of mRNA and dystrophin expression in DMD patients three months after myoblast transfer. Neuromuscular Disorders. 1995;**5**(4):291-295

[75] Miller RG, Sharma KR, Pavlath GK, Gussoni E, Mynhier M, Yu P, et al. Myoblast implantation in Duchenne muscular dystrophy: The San

Francisco study. Muscle & Nerve. 1997;**20**(4):469-478

[76] Mendell JR, Kissel JT, Amato AA, King W, Signore L, Prior TW, et al. Myoblast transfer in the treatment of Duchenne's muscular dystrophy. New England Journal of Medicine. 1995;**333**(13):832-838

[77] Gussoni E, Pavlath GK, Lanctot AM, Sharma KR, Miller RG, Steinman L, et al. Normal dystrophin transcripts detected in Duchenne muscular dystrophy patients after myoblast transplantation. Nature. 1992;**356**(6368):435-438

[78] Huard J, Bouchard JP, Roy R, Malouin F, Dansereau G, Labrecque C, et al. Human myoblast transplantation: Preliminary results of 4 cases. Muscle & Nerve. 1992;**15**(5):550-560

[79] Law PK, Goodwin TG, Fang Q, Duggirala V, Larkin C, Florendo JA, et al. Feasibility, safety, and efficacy of myoblast transfer therapy on Duchenne muscular dystrophy boys. Cell Transplant. 1992;**1**(2-3):235-244

[80] Tremblay JP, Malouin F, Roy R, Huard J, Bouchard JP, Satoh A, et al. Results of a triple blind clinical study of myoblast transplantations without immunosuppressive treatment In Young boys with Duchenne muscular dystrophy. Cell Transplant. 1993;**2**(2):99-112

[81] Montarras D, Morgan J, Collins C, Relaix F, Zaffran S, Cumano A, et al. Direct isolation of satellite cells for skeletal muscle regeneration. Science. 2005;**309**(5743):2064-2067

[82] Mouly V, Aamiri A, Périé S, Mamchaoui K, Barani A, Bigot A, et al. Myoblast transfer therapy: Is there any light at the end of the tunnel? Acta Myologica. 2005;**24**(2):128-133

[83] Price FD, Kuroda K, Rudnicki MA. Stem cell based therapies to treat muscular dystrophy. Biochimica et Biophysica Acta (BBA) - Molecular Basis of Disease. 2007;**1772**(2):272-283

[84] Fan Y, Maley M, Beilharz M, Grounds M. Rapid death of injected myoblasts in myoblast transfer therapy. Muscle & Nerve. 1996;**19**(7):853-860

[85] Skuk D, Goulet M, Tremblay JP. Use of repeating dispensers to increase the efficiency of the intramuscular myogenic cell injection procedure. Cell Transplantation. 2006;**15**(7):659-663

[86] Cell Therapy of Duchenne Muscular Dystrophy by intra-arterial delivery of HLA-identical allogeneic mesoangioblasts. EudraCT number: 2011-000176-33 [Internet]. [cited 2018 Nov 6]. Available from: https://www.clinicaltrialsregister.eu/ctr-search/search?query=eudract_number%3A2011-000176-33

[87] Torrente Y, Belicchi M, Marchesi C, D'antona G, Cogiamanian F, Pisati F, et al. Autologous transplantation of muscle-derived CD133+ stem cells in Duchenne muscle patients. Cell Transplantation. 2007;**16**(6):563-577

[88] Yang XF, Xu YF, Zhang YB, Wang HM, Lü NW, Wu YX, et al. Functional improvement of patients with progressive muscular dystrophy by bone marrow and umbilical cord blood mesenchymal stem cell transplantations. Zhonghua Yi XueZaZhi. 2009;**89**(36):2552-2556

[89] Zhang C, Chen W, Xiao LL, Tan EX, Luo SK, Zheng D, et al. Allogeneic umbilical cord blood stem cell transplantation in Duchenne muscular dystrophy. Zhonghua Yi XueZaZhi. 2005;**85**(8):522-525

[90] Rajput BS, Chakrabarti SK, Dongare VS, Ramirez CM, Deb KD. Human umbilical cord mesenchymal stem cells in the treatment of Duchenne muscular dystrophy: Safety and feasibility study in India. Journal of Stem Cells. 2015;**10**(2):141-156

[91] Sharma A, Sane H, Badhe P, Gokulchandran N, Kulkarni P, Lohiya M, et al. A clinical study shows safety and efficacy of autologous bone marrow mononuclear cell therapy to improve quality of life in muscular dystrophy patients. Cell Transplantation. 2013;**22**(1_suppl):127-138

[92] Sharma A, Sane H, Gokulchandra N, Sharan R, Paranjape A, Kulkarni P, et al. Effect of cellular therapy in progression of Becker's muscular dystrophy: A case study. European Journal of Translational Myology. 2016;**26**(1):61-66

[93] Sharma A, Badhe P, Sane H, Pai S, Kulkarni P, Bhagwanani K, et al. Halting of functional decline in a case of duchenne muscular dystrophy after cellular therapy |. International Journal of Recent Advances in Multidisciplinary Research (IJRAMR). 2017;**04**(02):2293-2297

[94] Sharma A, Gokulchandran N, Sane H, Lakhanpal V, Kulkarni P, et al. Stabilization Of Disease Progression In A Case Of Duchenne Muscular Dystrophy With Cellular Transplantation. Stem Cell Advances Research Therapy. 2017;**2017**:J112

[95] Sharma A, Sane H, Kulkarni P, Mehta D, Kaur J, Nandini G, et al. Effect of autologous bone marrow mononuclear cell transplantation coupled with rehabilitation in limb girdle muscular dystrophy – A case report. International Journal of Medical Research Health Sciences. 2016;**5**(12):1-7

[96] Alok S, Amruta P, Ritu V, Hemangi S, Nandini G, et al. Functional improvements and musculoskeletal magnetic resonance imaging with spectroscopy changes following cell therapy in a case of limb girdle muscular dystrophy. International Journal of Cell Science & Molecular Biology. 2017;**2**(4):555595

[97] Sharma A, Gokulchandran N, Chopra G, Kulkarni P, Lohia M, Badhe P, et al. Administration of Autologous Bone Marrow-Derived Mononuclear Cells in children with incurable neurological disorders and injury is safe and improves their quality of life. Cell Transplant. 2012;**21**(1):S79-S90

[98] Sharma A, Sane H, Gokulchandran N, Gandhi S, Bhovad P, Khopkar D, et al. The role of cell transplantation in modifying the course of limb girdle muscular dystrophy: A longitudinal 5-year study. Degenerative Neurological and Neuromuscular Disease. 2015;**2015**(5):93-102

[99] Sharma A, Paranjape A, Sane H, Bhagawanani K, Gokulchandran N, Badhe P. Cellular transplantation alters the disease progression in Becker's muscular dystrophy. Case reports in transplantation. 2013;**2013**:909328

[100] Sharma A, Sane H, Paranjape A, Badhe P, Gokulchandran N, Jacob V. Effect of cellular therapy seen on musculoskeletal magnetic resonance imaging in a case of Becker's muscular dystrophy. Journal of Case Reports. 2013;**5**(2):440-447

[101] Sharma A, Sane H, Varghese R, Paranjape A, Nivins S, Inamdar S, et al. Potential benefits of serial cell transplantation in a case of Duchenne Muscular Dystrophy. Open Journal

of Clinical and Medical Case Report, 2018;4(4):1382

[102] Sharma A, Sane H, Kaur J, Gokulchandran N, Paranjape A, Yadav J, et al. Autologous bone marrow mononuclear cell transplantation improves function in a case of Becker's muscular dystrophy. American Based Research Journal. 2016;**5**(2):12

[103] Sharma A, Sane H, Paranjape A, Bhagawanani K, Gokulchandran N, Badhe P. Autologous bone marrow mononuclear cell transplantation in Duchenne muscular dystrophy – A case report. The American Journal of Case Reports. 2014;**2014**(15):128-134

[104] Sharma A, Kulkarni P, Chopra G, Gokulchandran N, Lohia M, Badhe P. Autologous bone marrow-derived mononuclear cell transplantation in Duchenne muscular dystrophy. Indian Journal of Clinical Practice. 2012;**23**(3):169-172

[105] Sharma A, Paranjape A, Sane H, Gokulchandran N, Sawant D, Shirke S, et al. Effect of cellular therapy in a case of limb girdle muscular dystrophy. International journal of current medical and. Pharmaceutical Research. 2017;**3**(09):2377-2381

[106] Dai A, Baspinar O, Yeşilyurt A, Sun E, Aydemir Çİ, Öztel ON, et al. Efficacy of stem cell therapy in ambulatory and nonambulatory children with Duchenne muscular dystrophy–phase I–II. Degenerative Neurological and Neuromuscular Disease. 2018;**8**:63

[107] Duzhar V, Radchenko V, Gozhenko A, Badiuk N. Duchenne muscular dystrophy: Treatment with fetal progenitor cell transplant. Pharmacology online. 2021;**3**:1225-1230

[108] McDonald CM, Marbán E, Hendrix S, Hogan N, Smith RR, Eagle M, et al. Repeated intravenous cardiosphere-derived cell therapy in late-stage Duchenne muscular dystrophy (HOPE-2): A multicentre, randomised, double-blind, placebo-controlled, phase 2 trial. The Lancet. 2022;**399**(10329):1049-1058

[109] Haas R, Murea S. The role of granulocyte colony-stimulating factor in mobilization and transplantation of peripheral blood progenitor and stem cells. Cytokines and Molecular Therapy. 1995;**1**(4):249-270 Erratum in: Cytokines Mol Ther 1996;2(1):136

[110] Eljaszewicz A, Sienkiewicz D, Grubczak K, Okurowska-Zawada B, Paszko-Patej G, Miklasz P, et al. Effect of periodic granulocyte colony-stimulating factor administration on endothelial progenitor cells and different monocyte subsets in pediatric patients with muscular dystrophies. Stem Cells International. 2016;**2016**:2650849

[111] Sienkiewicz D, Kułak W, Okurows Eljaszewiczka-Zawada B, Paszko-Patej G, Wojtkowski J, Sochoń K, et al. Efficacy and the safety of granulocyte colony-stimulating factor treatment in patients with muscular dystrophy: A non-randomized clinical trial. Frontiers in Neurology. 2017;**8**:566

[112] Mäkelä J, Ylitalo K, Lehtonen S, Dahlbacka S, Niemelä E, Kiviluoma K, et al. Bone marrow–derived mononuclear cell transplantation improves myocardial recovery by enhancing cellular recruitment and differentiation at the infarction site. The Journal of Thoracic and Cardiovascular Surgery. 2007;**134**(3):565-573

[113] Sienkiewicz D, Kulak W, Okurowska-Zawada B, Paszko-Patej G, Kawnik K. Duchenne muscular dystrophy: Current cell therapies. Therapeutic Advances in Neurological Disorders. 2015;**8**(4):166-177

[114] Agadi S, Shetty AK. Concise review: Prospects of bone marrow mononuclear cells and mesenchymal stem cells for treating status epilepticus and chronic epilepsy. Stem Cells. 2015;**33**(7):2093-2103

[115] Sanchez-Ramos JR. Neural cells derived from adult bone marrow and umbilical cord blood. Journal of Neuroscience Research. 2002;**69**(6):880-893

[116] LaBarge MA, Blau HM. Biological progression from adult bone marrow to Mononucleate muscle stem cell to multinucleate muscle fiber in response to injury. Cell. 2002;**111**(4):589-601

[117] Cuende N, Rico L, Herrera C. Concise review: Bone marrow mononuclear cells for the treatment of ischemic syndromes: Medicinal product or cell transplantation? Stem Cells Translational Medicine. 2012;**1**(5):403-408

[118] Massimiliano G, Zhiping Z, Aiguo N, Dzau VJ. Paracrine mechanisms in adult stem cell signaling and therapy. Circulation Research. 2008;**103**(11):1204-1219

[119] Burdon TJ, Paul A, Noiseux N, Prakash S, Shum-Tim D. Bone marrow stem cell derived paracrine factors for regenerative medicine: current perspectives and therapeutic potential. Bone Marrow Research. 2011;**2011**:207326

[120] Arahata K, Engel AG. Monoclonal antibody analysis of mononuclear cells in myopathies. IV: Cell-mediated cytotoxicity and muscle fiber necrosis. Annals of Neurology. 1988;**23**(2):168-173

[121] Ichim TE, Alexandrescu DT, Solano F, Lara F, Campion RDN, Paris E, et al. Mesenchymal stem cells as anti-inflammatories: Implications for treatment of Duchenne muscular dystrophy. Cellular Immunology. 2010;**260**(2):75-82

[122] Turturici G, Tinnirello R, Sconzo G, Geraci F. Extracellular membrane vesicles as a mechanism of cell-to-cell communication: Advantages and disadvantages. American Journal of Physiology-Cell Physiology. 2014;**306**(7):C621-C633

[123] Biancone L, Bruno S, Deregibus MC, Tetta C, Camussi G. Therapeutic potential of mesenchymal stem cell-derived microvesicles. Nephrology, Dialysis, Transplantation. 2012;**27**(8):3037-3042

[124] Dastur DK, Razzak ZA. Possible neurogenic factor in muscular dystrophy: Its similarity to denervation atrophy. Journal of Neurology, Neurosurgery & Psychiatry. 1973;**36**(3):399-410

[125] Cerri S, Greco R, Levandis G, Ghezzi C, Mangione AS, Fuzzati-Armentero M-T, et al. Intracarotid infusion of mesenchymal stem cells in an animal model of Parkinson's disease, focusing on cell distribution and neuroprotective and behavioral effects. Stem Cells Translational Medicine. 2015;**4**(9):1073-1085

[126] Fischer UM, Harting MT, Jimenez F, Monzon-Posadas WO, Xue H, Savitz SI, et al. Pulmonary passage is a major obstacle for intravenous stem cell delivery: The pulmonary first-pass effect. Stem Cells and Development. 2008;**18**(5):683-692

[127] Palermo AT, Labarge MA, Doyonnas R, Pomerantz J, Blau HM. Bone marrow contribution to skeletal muscle: A physiological response to stress. Developmental Biology. 2005;**279**(2):336-344

[128] Christov C, Chrétien F, Abou-Khalil R, Bassez G, Vallet G, Authier F-J, et al. Muscle satellite cells and endothelial cells: Close neighbors and privileged partners. Molecular Biology of the Cell. 2007;**18**(4):1397-1409

[129] Germani A, Di Carlo A, Mangoni A, Straino S, Giacinti C, Turrini P, et al. Vascular endothelial growth factor modulates skeletal myoblast function. The American Journal of Pathology. 2003;**163**(4):1417-1428

[130] Sayers SP. The role of exercise as a therapy for children with Duchenne muscular dystrophy. Pediatric Exercise Science. 2000;**12**(1):23-33

[131] Gordon BS, Lowe DA, Kostek MC. Exercise increases utrophin protein expression in the mdx mouse model of Duchenne muscular dystrophy. Muscle & Nerve. 2014;**49**(6):915-918

[132] Simões GF, Benitez SU, Oliveira AL. Granulocyte colony-stimulating factor (G-CSF) positive effects on muscle fiber degeneration and gait recovery after nerve lesion in MDX mice. Brain and Behavior: A Cognitive Neuroscience Perspective. 2014;**4**(5):738-753

[133] Hayashiji N, Yuasa S, Miyagoe-Suzuki Y, et al. G-CSF supports long-term muscle regeneration in mouse models of muscular dystrophy. Nature Communications. 2015;**6**:6745

[134] Capoccia BJ, Shepherd RM, Link DC. G-CSF and AMD3100 mobilize monocytes into the blood that stimulate angiogenesis *in vivo* through a paracrine mechanism. Blood. 2006;**108**(7):2438-2445

[135] Hornby NL, Drees R, Harron R, Chang R, Wells DJ, Piercy RJ. Musculoskeletal magnetic resonance imaging in the DE50-MD dog model of Duchenne muscular dystrophy. Neuromuscular Disorders. 2021;**31**(8):736-751

[136] Díaz-Manera J, Llauger J, Gallardo E, Illa I. Muscle MRI in muscular dystrophies. Acta Myologica. 2015;**34**(2-3):95-108

[137] Barp A, Bello L, Caumo L, Campadello P, Semplicini C, Lazzarotto A, et al. Muscle MRI and functional outcome measures in Becker muscular dystrophy. Scientific Reports. 2017;**7**(1):16060

[138] Mazzone ES, Pane M, Sormani MP, Scalise R, Berardinelli A, Messina S, et al. 24 month longitudinal data in ambulant boys with Duchenne muscular dystrophy. PLoS One. 2013;**8**(1):e52512

[139] Kim HK, Merrow AC, Shiraj S, et al. Analysis of fatty infiltration and inflammation of the pelvic and thigh muscles in boys with Duchenne muscular dystrophy (DMD): Grading of disease involvement on MR imaging and correlation with clinical assessments. Pediatric Radiology. 2013;**43**(10):1327-1335

[140] Lu Y-M, Lue Y-J. Strength and functional measurement for patients with muscular dystrophy. In: Hegde M, Ankala A, editors. Muscular Dystrophy. Shanghai, China: London, UKInTech; 2012. pp. 321-331 [Internet]. [cited 2018 Nov 12]. Available from: https://www.intechopen.com/books/muscular-dystrophy/strength-decrease-pattern-and-functional-measurement-for-patients-with-muscular-dystrophy

[141] Steffensen BF, Lyager S, Werge B, Rahbek J, Mattsson E. Physical capacity in non-ambulatory people with Duchenne muscular dystrophy or spinal muscular atrophy: A longitudinal study. Developmental Medicine and Child Neurology. 2002;**44**(9):623-632

[142] Nguyen TH, Conotte S, Belayew A, Declèves AE, Legrand A, Tassin A. Hypoxia and hypoxia-inducible factor signaling in muscular dystrophies: Cause and consequences. International Journal of Molecular Sciences. 2021;**22**(13):7220

[143] Memar MY, Yekani M, Alizadeh N, Baghi HB. Hyperbaric oxygen therapy: Antimicrobial mechanisms and clinical application for infections. Biomedicine & Pharmacotherapy. 2019;**109**:440-447

[144] Yamamoto N, Oyaizu T, Enomoto M, Horie M, Yuasa M, Okawa A, et al. VEGF and bFGF induction by nitric oxide is associated with hyperbaric oxygen-induced angiogenesis and muscle regeneration. Scientific Reports. 2020;**10**(1):1-3

[145] Horie M, Enomoto M, Shimoda M, Okawa A, Miyakawa S, Yagishita K. Enhancement of satellite cell differentiation and functional recovery in injured skeletal muscle by hyperbaric oxygen treatment. Journal of Applied Physiology. 2014;**116**(2):149-155

[146] Thom SR, Bhopale VM, Velazquez OC, Goldstein LJ, Thom LH, Buerk DG. Stem cell mobilization by hyperbaric oxygen. American Journal of Physiology. Heart and Circulatory Physiology. 2006;**290**(4):H1378-H1386

[147] Hu Q, Liang X, Chen D, Chen Y, Doycheva D, Tang J, et al. Delayed hyperbaric oxygen therapy promotes neurogenesis through reactive oxygen species/hypoxia-inducible factor-1α/β-catenin pathway in middle cerebral artery occlusion rats. Stroke. 2014;**45**(6):1807-1814

[148] Leitman M, Efrati S, Fuchs S, et al. The effect of hyperbaric oxygenation therapy on myocardial function. The International Journal of Cardiovascular Imaging. 2020;**36**:833-840

[149] Akkawi I. Ozone therapy for musculoskeletal disorders: Current concepts. Acta Bio Medica: Atenei Parmensis. 2020;**91**(4):e2020191

[150] Williams IA, Allen DG. The role of reactive oxygen species in the hearts of dystrophin-deficient mdx mice. American Journal of Physiology-Heart and Circulatory Physiology. 2007;**293**(3):H1969-H1977

[151] Grounds MD, Terrill JR, Al-Mshhdani BA, Duong MN, Radley-Crabb HG, Arthur PG. Biomarkers for Duchenne muscular dystrophy: Myonecrosis, inflammation and oxidative stress. Disease Models & Mechanisms. 2020;**13**(2):dmm043638

[152] Bocci V. Is ozone really a "wonder drug"? In: Ozone. Dordrecht: Springer; 2010. pp. 85-96

[153] Kim J, Sung DJ, Lee J. Therapeutic effectiveness of instrument-assisted soft tissue mobilization for soft tissue injury: Mechanisms and practical application. Journal of Exercise Rehabilitation. 2017;**13**(1):12

[154] Crane JD, Ogborn DI, Cupido C, Melov S, Hubbard A, Bourgeois JM, et al. Massage therapy attenuates inflammatory signaling after exercise-induced muscle damage. Science Translational Medicine. 2012;**4**(119):119ra13

[155] Carroll K, Yiu EM, Ryan MM, Kennedy RA, de Valle K. The effects of calf massage in boys with Duchenne muscular dystrophy: A prospective interventional study. Disability and Rehabilitation. 2021;**43**(26):3803-3809

[156] Melone MA, Peluso G, Petillo O, Galderisi U, Cotrufo R. Defective growth in vitro of Duchenne muscular dystrophy myoblasts: The molecular and biochemical basis.

Journal of Cellular Biochemistry. 2000;**76**(1):118-132

[157] Bouffard NA, Cutroneo KR, Badger GJ, White SL, Buttolph TR, Ehrlich HP, et al. Tissue stretch decreases soluble TGF-β1 and type-1 procollagen in mouse subcutaneous connective tissue: Evidence from ex vivo and in vivo models. Journal of Cellular Physiology. 2008;**214**(2):389-395

[158] Hunt ER, Confides AL, Abshire SM, Dupont-Versteegden EE, Butterfield TA. Massage increases satellite cell number independent of the age-associated alterations in sarcolemma permeability. Physiological Reports. 2019;**7**(17):e14200

Chapter 3

Perspective Chapter: Multiple Functions of *Fukutin*, the Gene Responsible for Fukuyama Congenital Muscular Dystrophy, Especially in the Central Nervous System

Tomoko Yamamoto, Yukinori Okamura, Ryota Tsukui, Yoichiro Kato, Hiromi Onizuka and Kenta Masui

Abstract

Fukuyama congenital muscular dystrophy (FCMD), accompanying central nervous system (CNS) and ocular anomalies, is the second common muscular dystrophy in Japan, and the responsible gene is *fukutin*. The lesions are mainly caused by fragile basement membrane/cell membrane due to hypoglycosylation of α-dystroglycan (α-DG), and astrocytes play a crucial role for CNS malformation. On the other hand, since fukutin is expressed almost ubiquitously, diverse functions of fukutin, besides the glycosylation of α-DG, can be considered. As for the CNS, fukutin possibly upregulates cyclin D1 expression as a cofactor of activator protein-1 in astrocytoma. Moreover, fukutin may be involved in the phosphorylation of tau, one of the key proteins of dementia represented by Alzheimer's disease, in glutamatergic neurons. A presynaptic function in GABAergic neurons is also suggested. Owing to the recent advances of molecular and biochemical techniques, new therapeutic strategies are under consideration, even for brain malformation, which begins to be formed during the first trimester *in utero*. Recovery of hypoglycosylation of α-DG supposed to be a main therapeutic target, but to know various functions and regulation systems of fukutin might be important for developing suitable therapies.

Keywords: fukutin, multifunction, cell proliferation, astrocyte, tau phosphorylation, glutamatergic neuron, presynaptic function, GABAergic neuron

1. Introduction

Fukuyama congenital muscular dystrophy (FCMD), an autosomal recessive disease firstly reported by Fukuyama et al. in 1960 [1], is the second common muscular dystrophy in Japan [2]. It is one of the muscular dystrophies accompanies central nervous system (CNS) and ocular anomalies and is included in α-dystroglycanopathy [3, 4]. The responsible gene is *fukutin* [5]. α-dystroglycan (α-DG), a glycoprotein and a component of dystrophin-glycoprotein complex at the cell/basement membrane, binds to some basement membrane proteins, such as laminin-α2, neurexin-α, and agrin [4, 6]. The sugar chain works as a receptor [4, 6]. The expression is not only in the skeletal muscle but also in the CNS [7] and other organs [8]. Hypoglycosylation of α-DG causes fragile basement membrane, which is considered for the major pathogenesis of α-dystroglycanopathy. Several proteins including fukutin are involved in the glycosylation of α-DG [4, 6]. Fukutin has a function of ribitol 5-phosphate (Rbo5P) transferase that transfers Rbo5P from cytidine diphosphate-Rbo to α-DG [9]. α-DG is hypoglycosylated in the skeletal and cardiac muscles of FCMD patients [10]. Like α-DG, fukutin is expressed in various organs, almost ubiquitously [5, 8]. Diverse functions of fukutin can be suggested. To know these functions seems helpful not only for better understanding of FCMD pathology, but also for developing new therapeutic strategies. In this chapter, several intriguing roles of fukutin in the CNS are presented.

2. Fukutin gene

Fukutin is localized on chromosome 9q31 and encodes a 461-amino-acid protein [5]. The mRNA of 7349 bp contains an open reading frame of 1383 bp, composed of 10 exons, and a long 3′-untranslated region [5]. Alternative splicing has been found [11]. In FCMD, a common genetic mutation is a retro-transposal insertion of about 3000 bp into the 3′-untranslated region, called founder haplotype [5], but other mutations have been reported [11]. Mutations heavily affecting the coding protein may provoke a severe phenotype resembling Walker-Warburg syndrome [12–14], while those influencing lightly may cause mild phenotypes like limb girdle muscular dystrophy [12, 15, 16].

3. Clinicopathological characteristics of FCMD

Generally, FCMD patients are born as floppy infants, and peak motor function is achieved around 5 years old [2]. Patients usually die before 20 years old, but milder cases may live around 30 years old. Besides muscular dystrophy of the skeletal muscle, cardiac involvement is known. As clinical manifestations of the CNS lesion, mental retardation is observed, and more than 50% of patients show seizures. Ophthalmologic symptoms, such as myopia and abnormal eye movements, can be seen.

The CNS lesion of FCMD is represented by cobblestone lissencephaly, in other words polymicrogyria, of the cerebrum and cerebellum in post-natal cases [17, 18] (**Figure 1**). Abnormalities in the spinal cord may be found, especially in severe cases [19]. In the cerebrum and cerebellum of fetal cases, the glia limitans, covered with the basement membrane of the brain surface, is disrupted [20, 21]. In the cerebrum, overmigration of glioneuronal tissues through disruptions is obvious (**Figure 1**). The basement membrane/cell membrane at the glia limitans is abnormal, electron microscopically [21, 22]. Immunoreaction against anti-glycosylated α-DG [19] and laminin-α2 [23] antibodies is decreased at the glia limitans.

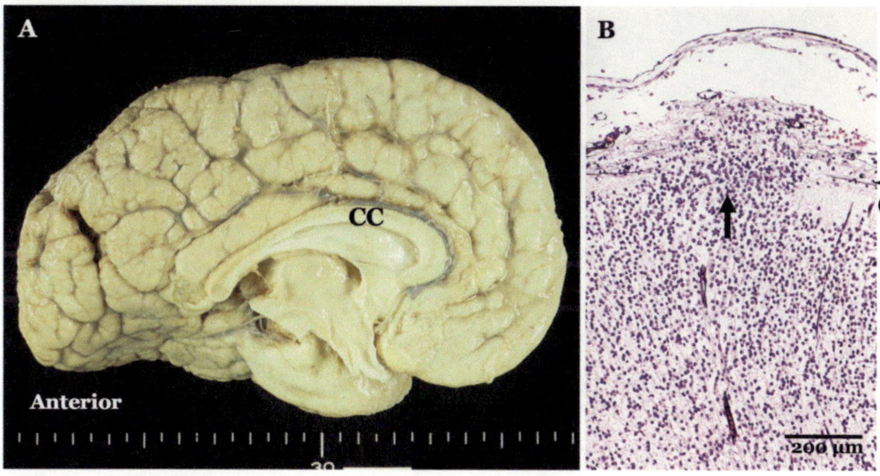

Figure 1.
Cerebral lesions of FCMD patients. A) Medial view of the cerebrum of 2-year-old case. Polymicrogyri are observed in the cortex. The corpus callosum looks normal. B) Cortical lesion of a fetus of 16 weeks of the gestation. Glioneuronal tissues overmigrate through a defect of glia limitans (arrow, periodic acid-methenamine-silver staining). CC: Corpus callosum, GL: Glia limitans.

4. Functions of fukutin in astrocytes

4.1 Functions related to the glycosylation of α-DG

The major pathogenesis of the polymicrogyria of FCMD is considered to be a fragile basement membrane due to hypoglycosylation of α-DG, which causes the disruption of the glia limitans [19]. Disruptions are already detectable in a fetus of 16 weeks of the gestation (**Figure 1**). Since astrocytes, expressing both α-DG [24] and fukutin [25], form the glia limitans, astrocytes are mainly involved in the pathogenesis of CNS lesions of FCMD [19]. The cerebrum and cerebellum show different histological appearances in polymicrogyria, owing to the difference of their structures, components, and ways of neuronal migration. In post-natal FCMD cases, the cerebral surface is continuous, exhibiting marked superficial gliosis with obvious elongation of astrocytic endfeet [19]. After maturation, astrocytes may be able to compensate the fragile basement membrane/cell membrane by reactive gliosis.

4.2 Functions other than the glycosylation of α-DG: relation to cell proliferation

In astrocytes, involvement in the glycosylation of α-DG is the most important role for the pathogenesis of CNS lesions of FCMD. However, other function of fukutin has been found, regarding the regulation of cell proliferation. On an astrocytoma cell line (1321 N1) highly expressing cyclin D1, cell proliferation and expression of cyclin D1 are decreased by suppression of fukutin and increased by overexpression (**Figure 2**) [26]. Cyclin D1, one of the proteins controlling the cell cycle, facilitates cells entering into the S phage of cell cycle for cell proliferation, and its expression is regulated by various transcription factors [27]. In the promoter area of cyclin D1, there are multiple binding sites for each transcription factor, including activator protein-1 (AP-1) [27]. It has been found that a complex

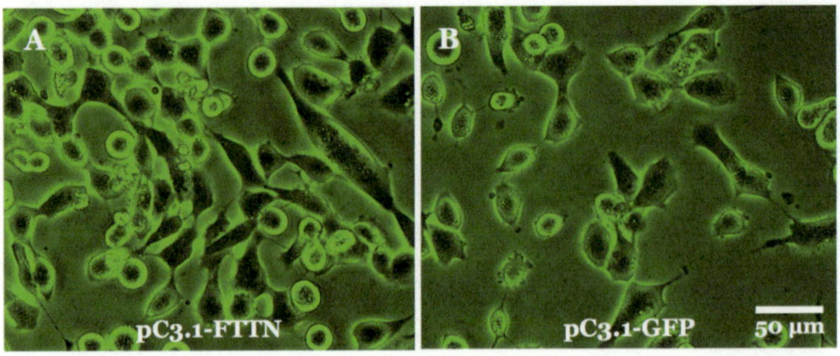

Figure 2.
Cell proliferation of astrocytoma cells (1321 N1) after transfection of fukutin. Cells increase in number with transfection of pC3.1-FKTN (a), compared with those with pC3.1-GFP (B). FKTN: Fukutin.

containing fukutin protein binds to the AP-1 binding site of cyclin D1 and fukutin protein and AP-1 are co-localized [26]. Fukutin can take part in the transcription regulation of cyclin D1 as a cofactor of AP-1, independent from the glycosylation of α-DG [26].

Astrocytes play a variety of roles to maintain the function of CNS properly, among which tissue repair is included. Activated astrocytes proliferate and migrate to repair damaged areas [28]. Given that fukutin is involved in the cell proliferation, a loss of fukutin in astrocytes might influence to wound healing in the CNS of FCMD patients, although studies have not been performed from this point of view to the author's knowledge. Apart from the pathogenesis of FCMD, it might be intriguing to investigate about fukutin on the standpoint of cell proliferation of astrocytoma. Fukutin might act as a cofactor of some other transcription factors besides AP-1.

5. Functions of fukutin in neurons

5.1 Functions in immature neurons

Although astrocytes are considered to play a crucial role to form the CNS lesions of FCMD, fukutin is also expressed in immature and mature neurons [25, 29]. In the cerebrum, immature neurons migrate from the ventricular zone to the cortical plate along with cytoplasmic processes of radial glia during the early fetal period [30, 31]. The migration is almost completed by 20–24 weeks of gestation [31]. Extracellular matrix proteins such as laminin and agrin are indispensable for the attachment of immature neurons and cytoplasmic processes of radial glia [32]. Since the sugar chain of α-DG is a receptor of such extracellular matrix proteins [4, 6], the glycosylated α-DG seems necessary for the neuronal migration [33]. Neurons begin to differentiate after settling to the proper place of the cerebral cortex [31]. Fukutin expression in immature neurons seems reasonable for the neuronal migration, smoothly interacting with radial glial fibers while keeping immaturity [34]. Irregular distribution of immature neurons is observed in the severely affected area of the cerebrum of FCMD, indicating that migration arrest may be apparent when a function of fukutin is seriously damaged [19]. Compensation of fukutin function by other proteins may be more established in neurons than in astrocytes.

5.2 Functions of fukutin in mature neurons

5.2.1 Function in glutamatergic neurons, with relation to the phosphorylation of tau

Fukutin expression is decreased in mature neurons [34], but some functions must exist in mature neurons. In the brain of FCMD patients more than 20 years old, neurofibrillary tangles (NFTs) immunopositive for phosphorylated tau (p-tau) are predominantly observed in the cerebral cortex [35, 36]. In our adult case of FCMD, NFTs are exclusively observed in areas showing polymicrogyria, and not found in the occipital robe showing almost normal appearance. In the CNS, there are excitatory and inhibitory neurons. The majority of neurons that constitute the cerebral cortex are excitatory/glutamatergic neurons, using glutamate as neurotransmitter, and the rests are inhibitory neurons [30]. Among several types of inhibitory neurons, neurons using γ-aminobutyric acid (GABA) as a neurotransmitter, GABAergic neurons, are a main component in the cerebral cortex [30]. GABA is synthesized from glutamate by glutamate decarboxylase (GAD) [37], which is used as a marker of GABAergic neurons. On immunohistochemical examination of the cerebrum of FCMD cases, neurons containing p-tau-positive NFT do not express GAD. NFTs are likely to be formed in excitatory neurons (**Figure 3**) [38]. Abnormal architectures of neurons derived from the disruption of glia limitans may be one of the factors to give rise to NFTs, considering from the distribution of neurons containing NFT. On the other hand, it is imaginable that fukutin itself is involved in the formation of NFTs.

In the adult CNS, there are six tau isoforms, which are divided into three microtubule-binding repeat (3R) and four microtubule-binding repeat (4R), depending on the absence or existence of exon 10 [39, 40]. There are various neurodegenerative diseases exhibiting p-tau-positive inclusions, so-called tauopathy. Three types of p-tau accumulation are known: 3R + 4R tauopathy, in which inclusions contain 3R and 4R tau, is represented by Alzheimer's disease; 3R tauopathy represented by Pick's disease; 4R tauopathy represented by corticobasal degeneration [39]. On FCMD, Western blotting [36] and immunohistochemical examination reveal both 4R and 3R tau in the diseased brain (**Figure 3**). There is something common on formation of p-tau-positive NFTs in FCMD and Alzheimer's disease. However, the distribution of NFTs is somewhat different. Alzheimer's disease shows NFTs predominantly distributed in

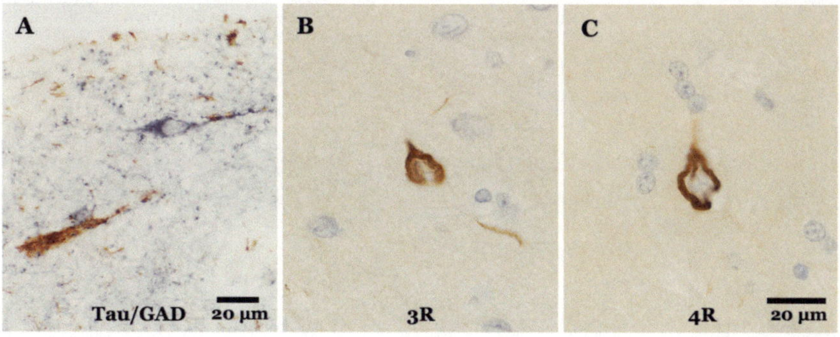

Figure 3.
Immunohistochemistry on the cerebrum of a 27-year-old FCMD patient. On double-immunohistochemical staining, p-tau (brown)-positive NFT is not formed in a glutamate decarboxylase (purple)-positive neuron (A). NFT is positive for both 3R tau (B) and 4R tau (C). NFT: Neurofibrillary tangle, GAD: Glutamate decarboxylase, 3R: Three microtubule-binding repeats, 4R: Four microtubule-binding repeats.

the limbic system and in the cerebral cortex, accompanying with senile plaques [41]. In contrast, NFTs are tended to be more in the cerebral cortex, and senile plaques are not found in FCMD. Different pathogenesis can be assumed.

Many molecules are involved in the phosphorylation of tau. One of the representative proteins is glycogen synthase kinase-3 (GSK-3β) [42]. Using neuroblastoma cell lines, we have found that the phosphorylation of both tau and GSK-3β is augmented by suppression of fukutin and is reduced by overexpression of fukutin [38]. Moreover, fukutin, tau, and GSK-3β are suggested to form a complex (**Figure 4**) [38]. Fukutin is possibly involved in the phosphorylation of tau, mediated by GSK-3β, which appears to be independent from the glycosylation of α-DG. It is likely that on glutamatergic neurons of the FCMD cerebrum, loss of fukutin accelerates the phosphorylation of tau, which may be augmented by abnormal network of neurons. Implication of GSK-3β is considered for this phosphorylation. However, GSK-3β is involved in the

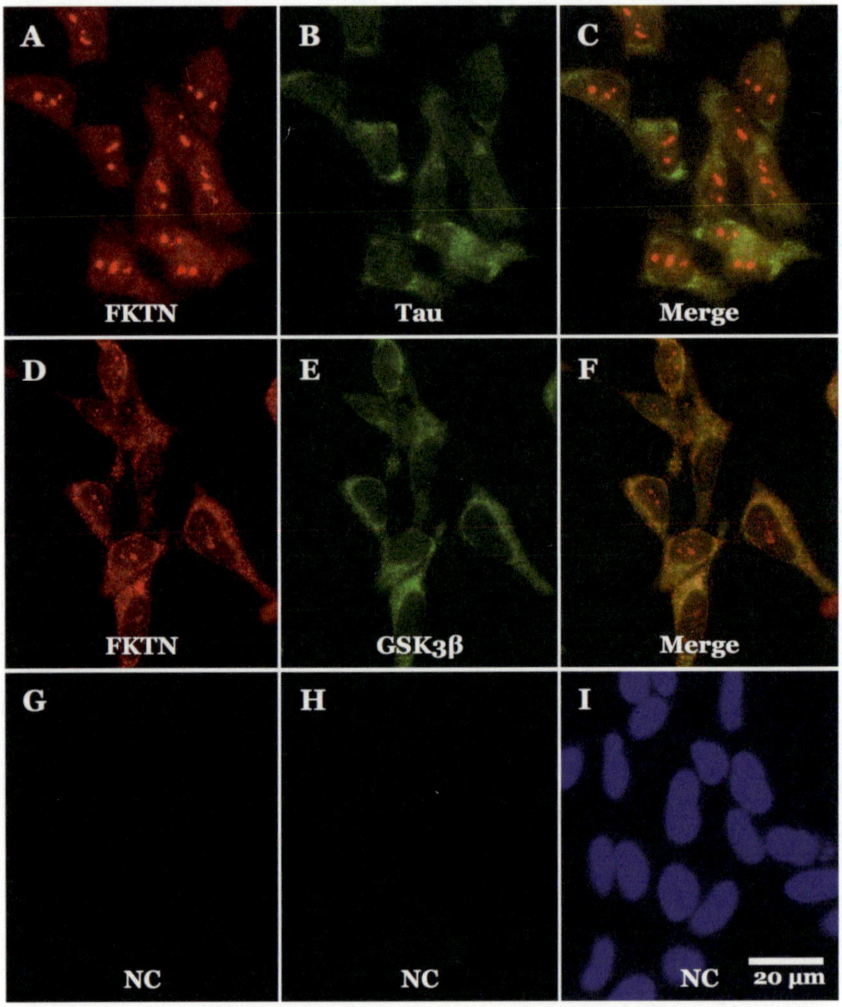

Figure 4.
Double-immunocytochemical staining on neuroblastoma cells (SH-SY5Y). Fukutin and tau are co-localized (A-C). Fukutin and glycogen synthase kinase-3 show similar localization (D-F). No immunoreaction is observed in negative controls (G-I). FKTN: Fukutin, GSK-3β: Glycogen synthase kinase-3 β.

abnormal accumulation of amyloid-β as well, a main component of senile plaque [42, 43]. Further studies are required to elucidate the mechanism between fukutin and tau phosphorylation.

5.2.2 Function in GABAergic neurons, with relation to the synaptic function

In the cerebrum of our adult FCMD patient, immunoreaction against anti-GAD antibody is increased [38]. Several factors can be postulated for the explanation, e.g., compensation toward hyperactivities of glutamatergic neurons, reaction against abnormal postsynaptic or presynaptic functions, etc. It is curious to know whether fukutin itself directly implicated in this phenomenon or not. A loss of fukutin appears to trigger the increase of GAD, because the increase is observed throughout the cerebral cortex, including the occipital robe showing almost normal histological appearance [38]. The dystrophin-dystroglycan complex (DGC) is existed in the postsynapse, and postsynaptic function of α-DG is well known [6, 44]. In contrast, studies about presynaptic functions of the DGC are not so many, but the DGC exists in the presynapse of GABAergic neurons [45]. On neuroblastoma cell lines, fluorescence immunocytochemistry has revealed that expression GAD is increased by suppression of fukutin and decreased by overexpression of fukutin [38]. Co-localization of fukutin, GAD, and synaptophysin is also suggested (**Figure 5**) [38]. Since synaptophysin is a component of presynaptic vesicle [46], co-localization of fukutin and synaptophysin supports presynaptic function of fukutin. From the existence of the DGC at the presynapse, increase of GAD in GABAergic neurons might result from the decreased glycosylation of α-DG, but co-localization of fukutin and GAD might indicate a direct involvement of fukutin.

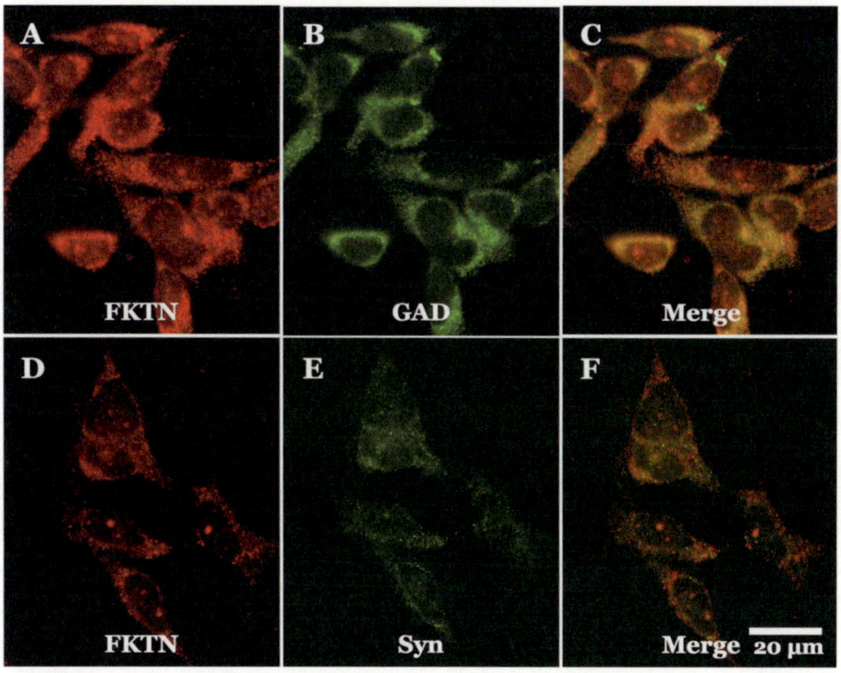

Figure 5.
Double- immunocytochemical staining on neuroblastoma cells (SH-SY5Y). Fukutin and glutamate decarboxylase are co-localized (A-C). Co-localization is also observed between fukutin and synaptophysin (D-F). FKTN: Fukutin, GAD: Glutamate decarboxylase, Syn: Synaptophysin.

6. Future perspectives

In addition to the glycosylation of α-DG, fukutin can contribute at least to cell proliferation, tau phosphorylation, and presynaptic function. The Golgi apparatus is considered to be a major subcellular localization [5, 47], because fukutin is involved in the glycosylation of α-DG. However, PSORT II prediction favors localizations of fukutin in the cytoplasm, mitochondria and nucleus rather than the Golgi apparatus. This prediction matches the findings presented in this chapter and suggests more unknown functions of fukutin.

With regard to the phosphorylation of tau, a relation between fukutin and microtubules can be assumed. Tau is a microtubule-binding protein to stabilize microtubules. Phosphorylated tau proteins that cannot bind to the microtubules are accumulated in the cytoplasm, resulting in NFTs [40]. Fukutin could be involved in the stabilization of microtubules by suppressing the phosphorylation of tau. When fukutin is knocked down on neuroblastoma cell lines, cytoplasmic processes are elongated (**Figure 6**) [34]. Elongation of cytoplasmic processes is also observed in fukutin-suppressed astrocytoma cells [48]. Astrocytes express tau, and astrocytic tau pathology has been reported [49]. It has been shown that overexpression of tau disturbs movements of kinesin, one of the representative molecular motors, and tau-stable cells exhibit rather round appearances [50]. Fukutin might relate to functions of microtubules via tau phosphorylation, not only influencing their stabilization but also affecting movements of molecular motors and cell morphology. A relation between fukutin and microtubules is proposed in cardiomyocytes as well [51]. To study more about the relation between fukutin and microtubules appears interesting.

To mention more about glial cells, there are four major types of glial cells in the CNS; astrocyte, oligodendrocyte, microglia, and ependymal cell. Functions of fukutin in astrocytes are indispensable for the pathogenesis of the CNS lesion of FCMD, while functions in other glial cells have not been elucidated. There are only a few observations suggesting functions of fukutin in oligodendrocytes. The cerebral white matter of FCMD exhibits dysmyelination [52], and fukutin-deficient chimera mice show loss of myelination in the peripheral nerve [53]. On microglia and ependymal cells, investigations relating to fukutin have not been found in English literatures to the authors' knowledge.

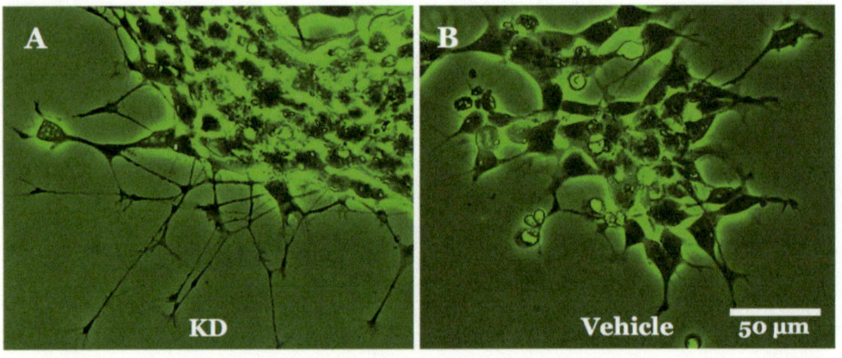

Figure 6.
Morphological alteration of neuroblastoma cells (IMR32) after suppression of fukutin. Elongation of cytoplasmic processes is conspicuous on cells with suppression of fukutin (A), compared with control cells (B). KD: Knockdown of fukutin.

As for therapies of FCMD, in addition to conventional treatments, efficacy of steroids [54] and rapamycin [55] has been suggested for muscular dystrophy. A retro-transposal insertion in the 3′-untranslated region of *fukutin* provokes pathogenic exon-trapping, resulting in a production of abnormal fukutin protein [56]. Treatment of antisense oligonucleotide can prevent this pathogenic exon trapping and restore normal fukutin production on human primary myotube obtained from FCMD patients and from FCMD model mice knocked in the retro-transposal insertion [56]. CDP-ribitol prodrug ameliorates muscular dystrophy in mice that lack *isoprenoid synthase domain-containing protein (ISPD)*, one of the causative genes of α-dystroglycanopathy [57]. Surprisingly, recent studies propose novel strategies toward brain malformation, despite the CNS and ocular anomalies begin to be formed during the first trimester *in utero*. Severe brain malformation of *Emx1-fukutin*-cKO mouse is prevented by delivery of fukutin into the brain at E12.5 [58]. In a brain organoid model of FCMD, abnormal radial glial fiber migration is restored by Mannan-007 [59]. It is not easy to overcome a lot of difficulties to apply new molecular or gene-based therapies, especially to fetuses. Unexpected phenomena could happen. On developing new therapeutic strategies, especially of molecular level, a good knowledge about functions and regulation systems of fukutin seems necessary.

7. Conclusion

Fukutin is considered to be multifunctional. In the CNS, fukutin can be involved at least in the cell proliferation, tau phosphorylation, and presynaptic function, some of which seems independent from the glycosylation of α-DG. To see fukutin form various standpoints may be interesting and indispensable, not only for deep understanding of FCMD pathology but also for developing suitable therapies.

Acknowledgements

The authors are grateful to ex-professor of the Department of Pathology, Noriyuki Shibata for valuable comments, and to Mr. Mizuho Karita, Mr. Hideyuki Takeiri, Ms. Noriko Sakayori, Mr. Fumiaki Muramatsu, and Mr. Shuichi Iwasaki for their excellent technical assistances.

The authors declare no conflict of interest.

Author details

Tomoko Yamamoto[1,2]*, Yukinori Okamura[1,2], Ryota Tsukui[3], Yoichiro Kato[2], Hiromi Onizuka[1,2] and Kenta Masui[1,2]

1 Department of Surgical Pathology, Tokyo Women's Medical University, Tokyo, Japan

2 Division of Human Pathology and Pathological Neuroscience, Department of Pathology, Tokyo Women's Medical University, Tokyo, Japan

3 Department of Anesthesiology, Tokyo Women's Medical University, Tokyo, Japan

*Address all correspondence to: yamamoto.tomoko@twmu.ac.jp

IntechOpen

© 2022 The Author(s). Licensee IntechOpen. This chapter is distributed under the terms of the Creative Commons Attribution License (http://creativecommons.org/licenses/by/3.0), which permits unrestricted use, distribution, and reproduction in any medium, provided the original work is properly cited.

References

[1] Fukuyama Y, Kawazura M, Haruna H. A peculiar form of congenital progressive muscular dystrophy. Paediatria Universitatis Tokyo. 1960;**4**:5-8

[2] Osawa M, Sumida S, Suzuki N, Arai Y, Ikenaka H, Murasugi H, et al. Fukuyama type congenital progressive muscular dystrophy. In: Fukuyama Y, Osawa M, Saito K, editors. Congenital Muscular Dystrophies. Amsterdam: Elsevier; 1997. pp. 31-68

[3] Martin PT. The dystroglycanopathies: The new disorders of O- linked glycosylation. Seminars in Pediatric Neurology. 2005;**12**:152-158. DOI: 10.1016/j.spen.2005.10.003

[4] Schessl J, Zou Y, Bönnemann CG. Congenital muscular dystrophies and the extracellular matrix. Seminars in Pediatric Neurology. 2006;**13**:80-89. DOI: 10.1016/j.spen.2006.06.003

[5] Kobayashi K, Nakahori Y, Miyake M, Matsumura K, Kondo-Iida E, Nomura Y, et al. An ancient retro- transposal insertion causes Fukuyama-type congenital muscular dystrophy. Nature. 1998;**394**:388-392. DOI: 10.1038/28653

[6] Waite A, Tinsley CL, Locke M, Blake DJ. The neurobiology of the dystrophin-associated glycoprotein complex. Annals of Medicine. 2009;**41**:344-359. DOI: 10.1080/07853890802668522

[7] Moukhles H, Carbonetto S. Dystroglycan contributes to the formation of multiple dystrophin-like complexes in brain. Journal of Neurochemistry. 2001;**78**:824-834. DOI: 10.1046/j.1471-4159.2001.00466.x

[8] Saito Y, Yamamoto T, Ohtsuka-Tsurumi E, Oka A, Mizuguchi M, Itoh M, et al. Fukutin expression in mouse non-muscle somatic organs: Its relationship to the hypoglycosylation of α-dystroglycan in Fukuyama-type congenital muscular dystrophy. Brain & Development. 2004;**26**:469-479. DOI: 10.1016/j.braindev.2004.01.004

[9] Kanagawa M, Kobayashi K, Tajiri M, Manya H, Kuga A, Yamaguchi Y, et al. Identification of a post-translational modification with ribitol-phosphate and its defect in muscular dystrophy. Cell Reports. 2016;**14**:2209-2223. DOI: 10.1016/j.celrep.2016.02.017

[10] Hayashi YK, Ogawa M, Tagawa K, Noguchi S, Ishihara T, Nonaka I, et al. Selective deficiency of alpha-dystroglycan in Fukuyama-type congenital muscular dystrophy. Neurology. 2001;**57**:115-121. DOI: 10.1212/wnl.57.1.115

[11] Kobayashi K, Sasaki J, Kondo-Iida E, Fukuda Y, Kinoshita M, Sunada Y, et al. Structural organization, complete genomic sequences and mutational analyses of the Fukuyama-type congenital muscular dystrophy gene, fukutin. FEBS Letters. 2001;**489**:192-196. DOI: 10.1016/s0014-5793(01)02088-9

[12] Beltrán-Valero de Bernabé D, van Bokhoven H, van Beusekom E, Van den Akker W, Kant S, Dobyns WB, et al. A homozygous nonsense mutation in the fukutin gene causes a Walker-Warburg syndrome phenotype. Journal of Medical Genetics. 2003;**40**:845-848. DOI: 10.1136/jmg.40.11.845

[13] Godfrey C, Clement E, Mein R, Brockington M, Smith J, Talim B, et al. Refining genotypa-phenotype

correlations in muscular dystrophies with defective glycosylation of dystroglycan. Brain. 2007;**130**:2725-2735. DOI: 10.1093/brain/awm212

[14] Cotarelo RP, Valero MC, Prados B, Peña A, Rodríguez L, Fano O, et al. Two new patients bearing mutations in the fukutin gene confirm the relevance of this gene in Walker-Warburg syndrome. Clinical Genetics. 2008;**73**:139-145. DOI: 10.1111/j.1399-0004.2007.00936.x

[15] Godfrey C, Escolar D, Brockington M, Clement EM, Mein R, Jimenez-Mallebrera C, et al. *Fukutin* gene mutations in steroid-responsive limb girdle muscular dystrophy. Annals of Neurology. 2006;**60**:603-610. DOI: 10.1002/ana.21006

[16] Murakami T, Hayashi YK, Noguchi S, Ogawa M, Nonaka I, Tanabe Y, et al. Fukutin gene mutations cause dilated cardiomyopathy with minimal muscle weakness. Annals of Neurology. 2006;**60**:597-602. DOI: 10.1002/ana.20973

[17] Kamoshita S, Konishi Y, Segawa M, Fukuyama Y. Congenital muscular dystrophy as a disease of the central nervous system. Archives of Neurology. 1976;**33**:513-516. DOI: 10.1001/archneur.1976.00500070055011

[18] Takada K, Nakamura H, Tanaka J. Cortical dysplasia in congenital muscular dystrophy with central nervous system involvement (Fukuyama type). Journal of Neuropathology and Experimental Neurology. 1984;**43**:395-407. DOI: 10.1097/00005072-198407000-00005

[19] Yamamoto T, Shibata N, Saito Y, Osawa M, Kobayashi M. Functions of fukutin, a gene responsible for Fukuyama type congenital muscular dystrophy, in neuromuscular system and other somatic organs. Central Nervous System Agents in Medicinal Chemistry. 2010;**10**:169-179. DOI: 10.2174/187152410791196369

[20] Takada K, Nakamura H, Suzumori K, Ishikawa T, Sugiyama N. Cortical dysplasia in a 23-week fetus with Fukuyama congenital muscular dystrophy (FCMD). Acta Neuropathologica. 1987;**74**:300-306. DOI: 0.1007/BF00688196

[21] Yamamoto T, Toyoda C, Kobayashi M, Kondo E, Saito K, Osawa M. Pial-glial barrier abnormalities in fetuses with Fukuyama congenital muscular dystrophy. Brain & Development. 1997;**19**:35-42. DOI: 10.1016/s0387-7604(96)00056-3

[22] Yamamoto T, Shibata N, Kanazawa M, Kobayashi M, Komori T, Kondo E, et al. Early ultrastructural changes in the central nervous system in Fukuyama congenital muscular dystrophy. Ultrastructural Pathology. 1997;**21**:355-360. DOI: 10.3109/01913129709021933

[23] Yamamoto T, Shibata N, Kanazawa M, Kobayashi M, Komori T, Ikeya K, et al. Localization of laminin subunits in the central nervous system in Fukuyama congenital muscular dystrophy: An immunohistochemical investigation. Acta Neuropathologica. 1997;**94**:173-179. DOI: 10.1007/s004010050690

[24] Zaccaria ML, Di Tommaso F, Brancaccio A, Paggi P, Petrucci TC. Dystroglycan distribution in adult mouse brain: A light and electron microscopy study. Neuroscience. 2001;**104**:311-324. DOI: 10.1016/s0306-4522(01)00092-6

[25] Yamamoto T, Kato Y, Karita M, Takeiri H, Muramatsu F, Kobayashi M, et al. Fukutin expression in glial cells and neurons: Implication in the brain lesions of Fukuyama congenital muscular

dystrophy. Acta Neuropathologica. 2002;**104**:217-224. DOI: 10.1007/s00401-002-0542-8

[26] Okamura Y, Yamamoto T, Tsukui R, Kato Y, Shibata N. Fukutin protein participates in cell proliferation by enhancing cyclin D1 expression through binding to the transcription factor activator protein-1: An in vitro study. International Journal of Molecular Sciences. 2021;**22**:12153. DOI: org/10.3390/ijms222212153

[27] Guo Z, Hao X, Tan F-F, Pei X, Shang L-M, Jiang X, et al. The elements of human cyclin D1 promoter and regulation involved. Clinical Epigenetics. 2011;**2**:63-76. DOI: 10.1007/s13148-010-0018-y

[28] Lagos-Cabré R, Burgos-Bravo F, Avalos AM, Leyton L. Connexins in astrocyte migration. Frontiers in Pharmacology. 2019;**10**:1546. DOI: 10.3389/fphar.2019.01546

[29] Sasaki J, Ishikawa K, Kobayashi K, Kondo-Iida E, Fukayama M, Mizusawa H, et al. Neuronal expression of the fukutin gene. Human Molecular Genetics. 2000;**9**:3083-3090. DOI: 10.1093/hmg/9.20.3083

[30] Hevner RF. From radial glia to pyramidal-projection neuron. Transcription factor cascades in cerebral cortex development. Molecular Neurobiology. 2006;**33**:33-50. DOI: 10.1385/MN:33:1:033

[31] Larroche J-C. Development of the central nervous system. In: Developmental Pathology of the Neonate. Amsterdam: Excerpta Medica; 1977. pp. 319-353

[32] Porcionatto MA. The extracellular matrix provides directional cues for neuronal migration during cerebellar development. Brazilian Journal of Medical and Biological Research. 2006;**39**:313-320. DOI: 10.1590/s0100-879x2006000300001

[33] Qu Q. Smith FI : Alpha-dystroglycan interactions affect cerebellar granule neuron migration. Journal of Neuroscience Research. 2004;**76**:771-782. DOI: 10.1002/jnr.20129

[34] Hiroi A, Yamamoto T, Shibata N, Osawa M, Kobayashi M. Roles of fukutin, the gene responsible for Fukuyama-type congenital muscular dystrophy, in neurons: Possible involvement in synaptic function and neuronal migration. Acta Histochemica et Cytochemica. 2011;**44**:91-101. DOI: 10.1267/ahc.10045

[35] Tanaka J, Minamitani M, Takada K. Brain pathology in Fukuyama type congenital muscular dystrophy with special reference to the cortical dysplasia and the occurrence of neurofibrillary tangles. In: Fukuyama Y, Osawa M, Saito K, editors. Congenital Muscular Dystrophies. Amsterdam: Elsevier; 1997. pp. 189-197

[36] Saito Y, Motoyoshi Y, Kashima T, Izumiyama-Shimomura N, Toda T, Nakano I, et al. Unique Tauopathy in Fukuyama-type congenital muscular dystrophy. Journal of Neuropathology and Experimental Neurology. 2005;**64**:1118-1126. DOI: 10.1097/01.jnen.0000190069.10633.c2

[37] Martin DL, Rimvall K. Regulation of γ-aminobutyric acid synthesis in the brain. Journal of Neurochemistry. 1993;**60**:395-407. DOI: 10.1111/j.1471-4159.1993.tb03165.x

[38] Tsukui R, Yamamoto T, Okamura Y, Kato Y, Shibata N. Fukutin regulates tau phosphorylation and synaptic function: Novel properties of fukutin in neurons.

Neuropathology. 2022;**42**:28-39. DOI: 10.1111/neup.12797

[39] Goedert M. Tau filaments in neurodegenerative diseases. FEBS Letters. 2018;**592**:2383-2391. DOI: 10.1002/1873-3468.13108

[40] Noble W, Hanger DP, Miller CCJ, Lovestone S. The importance of tau phosphorylation for neurodegenerative diseases. Frontiers in Neurology. 2013;**4**:83. DOI: 10.3389/fneur.2013.00083

[41] Lane CA, Hardy J, Schott JM. Alzheimer's disease. European Journal of Neurology. 2018;**25**:59-70. DOI: 10.1111/ene.13439

[42] Sayas CL, Avila J. GSK-3 and tau: A key duet in Alzheimer's disease. Cell. 2021;**10**:721. DOI: 10.3390/cells10040721

[43] Lauretti E, Dincer O, Praticò D. Glycogen synthase kinase-3 signaling in Alzheimer's disease. Biochimica et Biophysica Acta (BBA)-Molecular Cell Research. 2020;**1867**:118664. DOI: 10.1016/j.bbamcr.2020.118664

[44] Moore SA, Saito F, Chen J, Michele DE, Henry MD, Messing A, et al. Deletion of brain dystroglycan recapitulates aspects of congenital muscular dystrophy. Nature. 2002;**418**:422-425. DOI: 10.1038/nature00838

[45] Lévi S, Grady RM, Henry MD, Campbell KP, Sanes JR, Craig AM. Dystroglycan is selectively associated with inhibitory GABAergic synapses but is dispensable for their differentiation. The Journal of Neuroscience. 2002;**22**:4274-4285. DOI: 10.1523/JNEUROSCI.22-11-04274.2002

[46] Wiedenmann B. Synaptophysin a widespread constituent of small neuroendocrine vesicles and a new tool in tumor diagnosis. Acta Oncologica. 1991;**30**:435-440. DOI: 10.3109/02841869109092398

[47] Tachikawa M, Kanagawa M, Yu C-C, Kobayashi K, Toda T. Mislocalization of fukutin protein by disease-causing missense mutations can be rescued with treatments directed at folding amelioration. The Journal of Biological Chemistry. 2012;**287**:8398-8406. DOI: 10.1074/jbc.M111.300905

[48] Yamamoto T, Kato Y, Hiroi A, Shibata N, Osawa M, Kobayashi M. Post-transcriptional regulation of fukutin in an astrocytoma cell line. International Journal of Experimental Pathology. 2012;**93**:46-55. DOI: 10.1111/j.1365-2613.2011.00799.x

[49] Kovacs GG, Robinson JL, Xie SX, Lee EB, Grossman M, Wolk DA, et al. Evaluating the patterns of aging-related tau Astrogliopathy unravels novel insights into brain aging and neurodegenerative diseases. Journal of Neuropathology and Experimental Neurology. 2017;**76**:270-288. DOI: 10.1093/jnen/nlx007

[50] Ebneth A, Godemann R, Stamer K, Illenberger S, Trinczek B, Mandelkow E-M, et al. Overexpression of tau protein inhibits kinesin-dependent trafficking of vesicles, mitochondria, and endoplasmic reticulum: Implications for Alzheimer's disease. The Journal of Cell Biology. 1998;**143**:777-794. DOI: 10.1083/jcb.143.3.777

[51] Ujihara Y, Kanagawa M, Mohri S, Takatsu S, Kobayashi K, Toda T, et al. Elimination of fukutin reveals cellular and molecular pathomechanisms in muscular dystrophy- associated heart failure. Nature Communications. 2019;**10**:5754. DOI: 10.1038/s41467-019-13623-2

[52] Kato T, Funahashi M, Matsui A, Takashima S, Suzuki Y. MRI of disseminated developmental dysmyelination in Fukuyama type of CMD. Pediatric Neurology. 2000;**23**:385-388. DOI: 10.1016/s0887-8994(00)00210-1

[53] Saito F, Masaki T, Saito Y, Nakamura A, Takeda S, Shimizu T. Toda, Matsumura K: Defective peripheral nerve myelination and neuromuscular junction formation in fukutin-deficient chimeric mice. Journal of Neurochemistry. 2007;**101**:1712-1722. DOI: 10.1111/j.1471-4159.2007.04462.x

[54] Murakami T, Sato T, Adachi M, Ishiguro K, Shichiji M, Tachimori H, et al. Efficacy of steroid therapy for Fukuyama congenital muscular dystrophy. Scientific Reports. 2021;**11**:24229. DOI: 10.1038/s41598-021-03781-z

[55] Foltz SJ, Luan J, Call JA, Patel A, Peissig KB, Fortunato MJ, et al. Four-week rapamycin treatment improves muscular dystrophy in a fukutin-deficient mouse model of dystroglycanopathy. Skeletal Muscle. 2016;**6**:20. DOI: 10.1186/s13395-016-0091-9

[56] Taniguchi-Ikeda M, Kobayashi K, Kanagawa M, Yu C, Mori K, Oda T, et al. Pathogenic exon-trapping by SVA retrotransposon and rescue in Fukuyama muscular dystrophy. Nature. 2011;**478**:127-131. DOI: 10.1038/nature10456

[57] Tokuoka H, Imae R, Nakashima H, Manya H, Masuda C, Hoshino S, et al. CDP-ribitol prodrug treatment ameliorates ISPD-deficient muscular dystrophy mouse model. Nature Communications. 2022;**14**(13):1847. DOI: 10.1038/s41467-022-29473-4

[58] Sudo A, Kanagawa M, Kondo M, Ito C, Kobayashi K, Endo M, et al. Temporal requirement of dystroglycan glycosylation during brain development and rescue of severe cortical dysplasia via gene delivery in the fetal stage. Human Molecular Genetics. 2018;**27**:1174-1185. DOI: 10.1093/hmg/ddy032

[59] Taniguchi-Ikeda M, Koyanagi-Aoi M, Maruyama T, Takaori T, Hosoya A, Tezuka H, et al. Restoration of the defect in radial glial fiber migration and cortical plate organization in a brain organoid model of Fukuyama muscular dystrophy. iScience. 2021;**24**:103140. DOI: 10.1016/j.isci.2021.103140

Chapter 4

The Potential Benefits of Drug-Repositioning in Muscular Dystrophies

Ioana Lambrescu, Emilia Manole, Laura Cristina Ceafalan and Gisela Gaina

Abstract

Muscular dystrophies (MDs) are a complex group of rare neuromuscular disorders caused by genetic mutations that progressively weaken the muscles, resulting in an increasing level of disability. The underlying cause of these conditions consists of mutations in the genes in charge of a person's muscle composition and functionality. MD has no cure, but medications and therapy can help control symptoms and slow the disease's progression. Effective treatments have yet to be developed, despite the identification of the genetic origins and a thorough knowledge of the pathophysiological alterations that these illnesses induce. In this scenario, there is an urgent need for novel therapeutic options for these severe illnesses, and drug repositioning might be one feasible answer. In other words, drug repositioning/repurposing is an accelerated method of developing novel pharmaceuticals since the new indication is based on previously accessible safety, pharmacokinetic, and manufacturing data. This is particularly crucial for individuals with life-threatening illnesses such as MDs, who cannot wait for a conventional medication development cycle. This chapter aims to review the challenges and opportunities of drug-repositioning in a variety of MDs to establish novel treatment approaches for these incurable diseases.

Keywords: muscular dystrophies, drug-repositioning, drug-repurposing, novel therapies, utrophin

1. Introduction

Muscular dystrophies (MDs) are a diverse array of hereditary muscle disorders defined by gradual weakening in the affected muscles [1]. Even among people with the same condition and genetic abnormalities, there may be differences in the age at which symptoms first appear, the severity of those symptoms, the rate at which they advance, the prognosis, and the most effective treatment [2]. In terms of epidemiology, each form of MD is rather uncommon, but these conditions account for a significant portion of the individuals who suffer from neuromuscular impairment [2].

Over the past decades, significant advancements have been achieved in the treatment of people who suffer from MD. This progress has been made possible by worldwide cooperation, increasing comprehension of the fundamental genetic mechanisms, and clinical consensus standards [3]. Therapeutic advancements have also expanded, first using mutation and gene-directed techniques, leading to commercially accessible medications targeting particular Duchenne muscular dystrophy (DMD) mutations [3]. Although there is real enthusiasm in the therapeutic area, it is crucial to remember that, since MDs are degenerative conditions, finding a permanent solution will be exceedingly difficult. Therefore, there is an urgent need to find and use innovative pharmacological treatments to enhance the clinical care of MD patients.

Drug repositioning, also known as pharmacological repurposing, is a process that may be used to find innovative therapeutic agents from the current drug molecules that the FDA has authorized for use in clinical settings [4]. Costs for novel treatments may be a significant barrier for researchers and patients in general and with rare illnesses in particular. This difficulty may be significantly addressed by experimenting with the usage of chemicals that were initially intended for other situations.

On average, the success rate of developing a new drug is only 2.01%. According to a report by the Eastern Research Group (ERG), it takes 10 to 15 years to generate a new therapeutic molecule [5]. Furthermore, traditional drug development processes generally include five phases, while drug repurposing only requires four (**Figure 1**) [6]. Researchers currently only require 1–2 years to uncover novel therapeutic targets, while it takes an average of 8 years to produce a repositioned medicine, thanks to the rapid growth of bioinformatics [7].

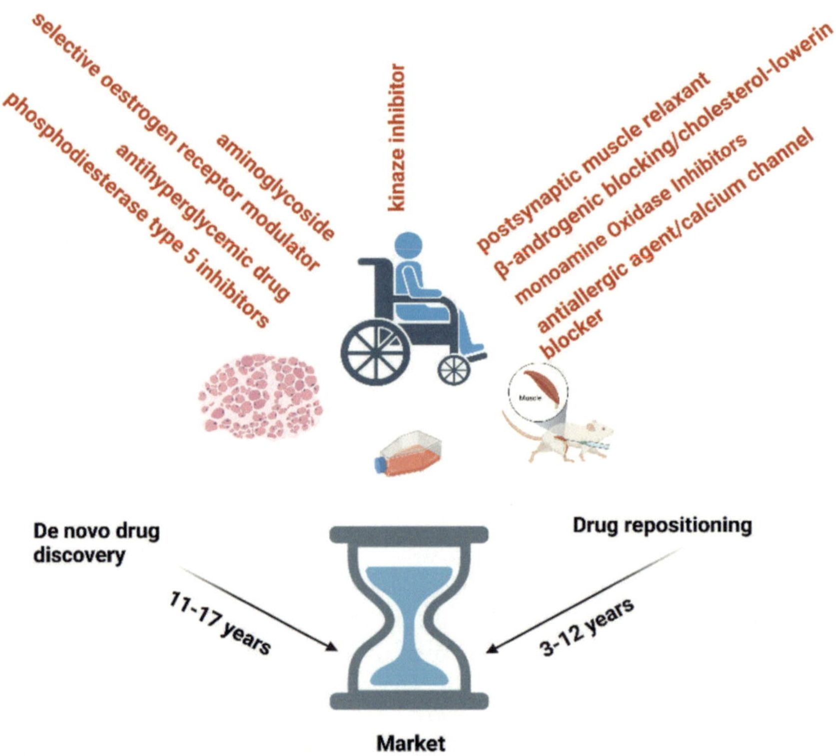

Figure 1.
Approaches for drug repurposing.

This chapter focuses on the most promising options for repositioning medications for three of the most prevalent forms of MDs: both in preclinical investigations and clinical trials.

2. DMD/BMD: showing old molecules how to accomplish new things

The X-linked muscle disorders known as dystrophinopathies include the muscular dystrophies Duchenne (DMD), Becker (BMD), and DMD-associated dilated cardiomyopathy (D). DMD, an X-linked recessive condition that mostly affects men, is characterized clinically by gradual muscular weakening and deterioration that initially affects proximal muscles [8]. The dystrophin gene (*DMD* gene), which is located on chromosome Xp21.2 and encodes for the dystrophin protein via its 79 exons, is the cause of DMD and BMD depending on the mutation [9]. Dystrophin is an essential component of the protein complex that via the cell membrane binds the cytoskeleton of a muscle fiber to the surrounding extracellular matrix, stabilizing it during muscle contraction [8]. A number of potentially useful therapy techniques have been created and studied using DMD animal models. Nevertheless, the results of clinical trials have been far less spectacular. Currently, there are no treatments that can reverse dystrophinopathies underlying etiology. Conventional therapies employing corticosteroids aim to relieve symptoms, but their long-term administration is linked with substantial side effects [10]. Regarding the concept of targeted therapy several approaches have been developed for restoring dystrophin, each customized to a specific type of mutation. Stop-codon read-through, exon skipping, vector-mediated gene therapy, and the emerging CRISPR/Cas9 gene editing are all promising strategies. However, in the context of these therapies, the initial enthusiasm is overshadowed by all the questions regarding treatment effect, safety, and financial burden [11]. Therefore, drug repositioning could be a cost and time-effective approach when it comes to a rare disease such as muscular dystrophy.

2.1 Targeting Utrophin a via repurposed drugs

Dystrophin's primary purpose in terms of its functional role is to forge a connection between the internal cytoskeletal actin network and the extracellular matrix. Consequently, this will ensure that the sarcolemma of muscle fibers retains its structural integrity [12, 13]. Utrophin, a paralogue of dystrophin, is a protein highly expressed in developing muscle [14]. To complete the connection from the cytoskeleton through the membrane and into the extracellular matrix, utrophin interacts with the dystrophin-associated protein complex [14]. Therefore, techniques based on targeting dystrophin or utrophin may be applied together in dystrophic muscles. There are two full transcription forms for utrophin. The neuromuscular junction (NMJ), tendon, choroid plexus, pia mater, and glomerulus all express utrophin A, whereas endothelial cells produce utrophin B [15]. Muscle-specific trans-factor known as eukaryotic elongation factor 1A2 (eEF1A2) was discovered to interact with utrophin A's 5'UTR, which is why eEF1A2 targeting might be a possible therapeutic approach for DMD patients [16].

In 2020, Peladeau and colleagues published an interesting study that aimed to identify FDA-approved drugs that acted on the eEF1A2-utrophin A pathway in *mdx* mice [17]. The *in vitro* and *in vivo* experiments focused on five leads: Acarbose, Betaxolol, Labetalol, Pravastatin, and Telbivudine. The authors found that the beta-androgenic blocking medication *Betaxolol* and the cholesterol-lowering medication *Pravastatin* were the most effective activators of both eEF1A2 and utrophin through its 5′UTR internal ribosome entry site. This observation was based on a 7-day drug treatment of transgenic mice harboring the bicistronic reporter construct containing the utrophin 5'UTR. Furthermore, muscle strength was increased, and both muscle fiber shape and sarcolemma integrity were improved after *mdx* mice were treated with these medicines for 4 weeks [17].

2.2 The monoamine oxidase inhibitors

Although the pathophysiological basis for DMD is yet unknown, oxidative stress and mitochondrial dysfunction are thought to be major contributors to the development of muscle injury [18–20]. In dystrophic muscles, the mitochondrial enzyme known as monoamine oxidase (MAO) is a key generator of reactive oxygen species (ROS). This mitochondrial enzyme has been researched extensively in the central nervous system [21]. In 2010, a group conducted by Menazza demonstrated that oxidative changes of myofibrillar proteins and cell death, which result in a notable decrease in contractile performance, are significantly influenced by MAO-dependent reactive oxygen species (ROS) buildup [21]. *Pargyline*, an inhibitor of both MAO isoforms, was introduced in the US and the UK in 1963 as an antihypertensive drug. This compound was also administered to dystrophic animals, resulting in a reduction in tropomyosin oxidation and an improvement in disease phenotype [21]. Nevertheless, Pargyline's clinical use has been halted due to its considerable adverse effects [22].

Safinamide is a potent and specific inhibitor of MAO-B, which is approved for the treatment of mid to late-stage fluctuating Parkinson's disease [23]. Since intracellular signaling requires a small amount of ROS, the specificity of MAO inhibition is a crucial element [24]. In 2018, Vitiello and colleagues analyzed the impact of safinamide on the skeletal muscle of *mdx* mice and cultured muscle cells obtained from DMD patients. Even after a brief (1 week) course of therapy, reducing MAO-B had a beneficial impact *in vivo*, indicating a mechanism lacking significant tissue remodeling. The reduction of reactive oxygen species (ROS) levels in the fibers of treated animals and the oxidative status of a critical component of the contractile apparatus (tropomyosin) has been confirmed by analysis of muscle sections taken from animals that were given safinamide. Given that *in vitro* cultures, the dystrophin gene is expressed in myotubes but not in myoblasts, the in vitro experiments showed that increased susceptibility to oxidative stress in dystrophic cells appeared to be independent of dystrophin expression [24].

The observation that MAO catalyzes catecholamine removal proves the potential benefit of MAO treatment in DMD [21]. Chronic diseases can be associated with an increased level of catecholamines and DMD patients make no exception to this rule, as an excess of urine catecholamine has been documented in connection to age and disease progression [25]. All of this information, along with the benefit of using MAO-B inhibitors to prevent the hypertensive crisis that MAO-A inhibitors might cause, makes safinamide a therapy with a safe profile capable of increasing muscle performance [24].

2.3 The selective estrogen receptor modulator

Tamoxifen, a selective estrogen receptor modulator, has been commonly used to treat breast cancer for decades [26]. Estrogen receptor alpha (ER), the target via which tamoxifen operates, is present in both skeletal and cardiac muscle [27, 28]. Numerous studies have shown that tamoxifen protects against contraction-induced membrane damage, controls calcium influx, reduces oxidative stress, and prevents fibrosis [29–32], which is why it was hypothesized that DMD patients could benefit from this drug. In 2013, Dorchies and colleagues published an interesting study that assessed the effect of tamoxifen on dystrophic muscle structure and function [33]. Compared to previous research on normal rodents, the effects observed in the current study were attained with tissue levels of TAM and its primary metabolites that were significantly smaller. A daily dose of 10 mg/kg/day delivered to mdx^{5Cv} mice for 15 months enhanced whole-body force, causing a change toward a slower phenotype [33].

The main DMD charity in the UK published a statement in July 2022 on preliminary data from the tamoxifen-DMD clinical case–control trial. The collaborating parties were disappointed to conclude that although patients receiving tamoxifen showed less disease progression, the differences between the tamoxifen and placebo group did not reach statistical significance [34]. For more DMD clinical trials please refer to **Table 1**.

2.4 Dantrolene—Then and now

Dantrolene sodium is a postsynaptic muscle relaxant that inhibits calcium release from the sarcoplasmic reticulum, reducing excitation-contraction coupling in muscle cells [35]. Since 1991, researchers have examined how this compound affects DMD, finding that it significantly lowers CK levels during the first year of treatment compared to age-matched historical controls [35]. Dantrolene is the agent of choice for treating and preventing malignant hyperthermia, a condition triggered by general anesthesia [36].

Exon skipping is a novel therapy that employs an antisense oligonucleotide (ASOs) customized to the patient's DNA mutation to target particular exons for exclusion from mRNA. As a result, the out-of-frame DMD mutation is converted to in-frame deletions, which might result in a partly functioning dystrophin protein [37]. Although 30% of patients may benefit from the existing exon skipping, most of the research on these therapies has focused on low-level dystrophin restoration (less than 6%) [38]. Due to differences in increased muscular function, across clinical studies small molecules were used to augment the effect of exon skipping. Dantolene's safety profile is already known due to its use in patients with DMD and malignant hyperthermia. This information, in conjunction with the fact that this drug reduced CK levels in both *mdx* mice and humans, raised the question of whether dantrolene can modulate exon skipping [35, 39]. Kendall and colleagues tried to answer this question by administering ASOs and dantrolene to *mdx* mice. The authors observed that DMD-directed ASOs and dantrolene cooperate to enhance targeted DMD exon skipping probably by interacting with specific molecular targets that subtly influence splicing activity. A further benefit of dantrolene is that it is effective independent of the specific ASO sequence, as seen by the enhancement of exon skipping activity for human exons 50 and 51 and mouse exon 23 [37]. In 2019, the group conducted by Berthelemy looked into the effects of dantrolene on skipping exons 44 and 45 in cultured myotubes from DMD patients' inducible directly reprogrammable myotubes (iDRMs) and induced pluripotent stem cells (iPSCs) [40]. In both exon 44 and 45 skip-amendable DMD cell models, the administration of dantrolene with the suitable ASOs raises the level of skipped mRNA compared with ASO alone. In patient-derived

Compound	Group	Original indication	Preclinical studies	Clinical trials
[Tamoxifen]	estrogen receptor modulator	breast cancer	10.1093/hmg/ddn151 10.1093/hmg/ddy258 10.1016/j.nmd.2021.09.003 10.1038/s41536-022-00214-x 10.1016/j.ajpath.2012.10.018 10.1085/jgp.202213081 10.1038/s41598-020-67,372-0 10.1089/scd.2016.0136 10.1038/mtm.2014.25 10.1371/journal.pone.0016184	NCT02835079 NCT03354039
Statins	HMG-CoA reductase inhibitor	reduce blood levels of low-density lipoprotein (LDL) cholesterol	10.3390/ijms23042016 10.1186/s13395-021-00273-3 10.3233/JND-200524 10.1038/s41467-020-15,971-w 10.14814/phy2.14018 10.1073/pnas.1509536112	—
Pargyline	Monoamine oxidase inhibitors	moderate to severe hypertension	10.1093/hmg/ddq339 10.1016/j.freeradbiomed.2014.07.006 10.3389/fphys.2018.01087 10.1038/nrn1883	—
Safinamide		Parkinson's disease		
Dantrolene sodium	postsynaptic muscle relaxant	malignant hyperthermia	10.1016/j.xcrm.2021.100298 10.1016/j.omtn.2019.09.020 10.1016/j.omnt.2018.02.002 10.1007/978-1-4939-8651-4_19 10.1126/scitranslmed.3005054	—
Metformin	biguanide	type 2 diabetes mellitus	10.15252/embr.202153955 10.1080/21655979.2021.1967029 10.3389/fphys.2021.642908 10.3389/fcell.2020.609493 10.1016/j.bcp.2018.04.022 10.1002/mus.24692	NCT02516085 NCT01995032
Tranilast			10.1186/1755-1536-7-1	10.1186/s13023-022-02352-3* 10.2169/internalmedicine.8651-16**

Compound	Group	Original indication	Preclinical studies	Clinical trials
Sildenafil	phosphodiesterase type 5 inhibitors	erectile dysfunction	10.1152/japplphysiol.00664.2018 10.1096/fj.201700249R 10.1093/hmg/ddt579 10.1093/hmg/dds415 10.1002/path.4054 10.1152/ajpheart.00522.2010 10.1073/pnas.1013077107	NCT01580501 NCT01168908 NCT01359670
Tadalafil	phosphodiesterase type 5 inhibitors	erectile dysfunction	10.1161/JAHA.116.003911 10.1002/jcp.25075 10.1371/journal.pone.0000806	NCT01580501 NCT05195775 NCT01359670 NCT01865084 10.1371/journal.pone.0232870 10.1002/mus.26736
Nintedanib	kinase inhibitor	idiopathic pulmonary fibrosis	10.1038/s41419-018-0792-6	—
Sunitinib	kinase inhibitor	gastrointestinal stromal tumor renal cell carcinoma well-differentiated pancreatic neuroendocrine tumors	10.1093/hmg/ddac042 10.1093/hmg/ddz044	—
Zidovudine	antiretroviral	HIV/AIDS	10.1186/s40478-018-0530-4	—
Streptomycin	aminoglycoside	bacterial infections	10.1152/ajpcell.000056.2011 10.1016/j.ajpath.2010.11.027 10.1371/journal.pone.00003644 10.1152/ajpheart.00688.2006 10.1016/j.nmd.2006.07.024 10.1113/jphysiol.2004.075275	—

Compound	Group	Original indication	Preclinical studies	Clinical trials
Gentamicin	aminoglycoside	bacterial infections	10.1073/pnas.2122004119 10.1093/nar/gkab194 10.1093/hmg/dds223 10.1248/bpb.34.712 10.1016/j.ejphar.2009.11.034 10.1111/j.1582-4934.2009.00718.x 10.1096/fj.08-115,618 10.1016/j.nbd.2008.07.009	NCT00451074 NCT00005574

**The study included DMD, BMD, and LGMD patients.*
***Pilot study.*

Table 1.
Examples of repurposed drugs for muscular dystrophies.

iDRM DMD myotube culture, dantrolene increases exon 44 skippings. Even though the improvement is small, it is still important because research shows that even small amounts of dystrophin can affect muscles [40].

2.5 Repositioning cardiological drugs

Dilated cardiomyopathy (DCM) is a severe consequence of DMD and one of the most important predictors of life expectancy [24]. In the context of this causality, it might be argued that therapy for the DCM serves as "repositioning." In DMD patients, **angiotensin-converting enzyme inhibitors** (ACEi) and **ß-blockers** (BBs) (and less often diuretics) are recommended for the reduction of peripheral circulatory resistance, blood volume, hyperadrenergic activation and oxygen consumption [24, 41, 42]. In addition, it is well known that BBs lower the incidence of potentially life-threatening arrhythmias initiated by foci of myocardial fibrosis [42]. Tamoxifen is another medication that has been demonstrated to impact the heart muscle significantly. The group conducted by Dorchies revealed that tamoxifen reduced cardiac fibrosis by 50% and positively impacted the diaphragm. As a result, there was a significant quantity of contractile tissue made accessible for respiratory function in the *mdx*^{5Cv} mouse model [33]. The question of whether or not these treatments qualify as repositioning drugs is less significant when viewed in the context of the fact that cardiovascular and respiratory disorders are unavoidable complications of DMD. It is for this reason that we have devoted a brief subchapter to discussing them.

Calcium is essential for muscular function, but its intracellular accumulation is toxic, triggering apoptosis. As the literature provides extensive research on the function of calcium in muscle injury, it is fair to speculate that calcium antagonists may be useful in DMD [43].

A Cochrane database of systematic reviews investigating the impact of calcium antagonists on muscular power and function in DMD was published by Phillips and Quinlivan in 2008 [44]. The authors conclude that although *verapamil* significantly increased muscular strength, it also caused several cardiac adverse effects [45]. Additionally, no significant differences in efficacy between *diltiazem, nifedipine*, and *flunarizine* were found in the remaining studies [44]. In 2009, Matsumura and colleagues published an interesting study that evaluated the effect of verapamil and diltiazem in *mdx* mice [46]. The dystrophic phenotype of *mdx* mice was improved as shown by a lower serum CK level and reduced muscle deterioration in the diaphragm. Moreover, between the two calcium antagonists, diltiazem seems to protect against muscle degeneration more effectively [46].

Nifedipine, another calcium channel blocker, was the main focus of a 2013 study by Altamirano [47]. The results add to the growing body of data indicating that the calcium level is high in *mdx* muscles and may be regulated by nifedipine. On *mdx* mice, this treatment resulted in a reduction in the basal ATP release from dystrophic fibers and a decreased prooxidative/apoptotic gene expression. Consequently, a reduced muscle injury was observed in *mdx* mice, as shown by a substantial decrease in serum CK and an improvement in muscular strength [47].

2.6 Metformin: A pleiotropic drug

As monotherapy or in combination with other medications, *metformin*, a biguanide, is now one of the most often prescribed drugs in the world for the treatment of type 2 diabetes (T2D) [48]. Metformin has a wide range of molecular mechanisms of action, which explain why it may be used to treat autoimmune illnesses, prevent cancer, and protect the cardiovascular system [49–51]. Pharmacological actions of metformin include a decrease of glucose and lipid production via inhibition of mitochondrial complex I (NADH: ubiquinone oxidoreductase) and activation of AMP-activated protein kinase (AMPK) [52]. In this context, it was natural for researchers and clinicians to be drawn to the possible use of this medication in MDs.

Metformin's potential to improve muscular fibrosis and strength was shown in mdx mice via non-AMPK-related pathways [53]. Another preclinical study led by Lai and colleagues hypothesized that metformin could downregulate different chemokines in MD mouse models [54]. Thus, in mdx mice, levels of CXCL12 (C–X–C motif chemokine ligand 12) both a glucocorticoid target and a differentially expressed gene and its receptor CXCR4 (C–X–C motif chemokine receptor 4) were increased. As a result of prednisone therapy, their concentration decreased considerably. Furthermore, CXCL12 and CXCR4 expression was similarly shown to be reduced in mdx mice after treatment with metformin, suggesting that this pathway may be an attractive therapeutic target for DMD [54].

As previously discussed, ASOs-mediated exon-skipping is a promising line of treatment for DMD patients. However, a significant obstacle to its therapeutic use is the poor systemic effectiveness, necessitating drugs that enhance ASOs' activity. Based on previous studies that demonstrated an improvement of phosphorodiamidate morpholino oligomer (PMO) delivery to peripheral muscle in mdx mice by intravenous administration of glycine, the group conducted by Lin analyzed the effect of oral glycine and metformin alongside PMO in dystrophin/utrophin double knock-out (DKO) mice [55]. Thus, without any toxicity that could be detected and with a life span extension, the scientists demonstrated improvements in the cardio-respiratory and skeletal systems and a phenotypic rescue in DKO mice [55].

Though widely administered in the T2D adult population it is important to mention that metformin has been tested in children and adolescents with neurogenic defects and muscle disorders [56]. In 2010, Casteels and colleagues reported that metformin is an insulin sensitizer capable of limiting weight gain and visceral adiposity in children with a neurogenic or myogenic motor deficit [56]. Thus, exploring the use of metformin as an additional therapy in a variety of illnesses has reached the clinical context of DMD. In 2019, Hafner and colleagues published the results of a randomized double-blind placebo-controlled parallel-group clinical trial that included 47 ambulant male children aged 6.5 to 10 years with DMD that received treatment with a combination of l-citrulline and metformin. Among ambulant patients with DMD, the co-treatment was not associated with an overall halting of the decline in motor function, although the stable subgroup of patients presented a decrease in motor function impairment [57]. Also, Metformin or L-citrulline supplementation in BMD patients results in notable antidromic changes in the arginine glycine amidinotransferase and guanidinoacetate methyltransferase pathways.

Metformin treatment has also been shown to be useful in congenital muscular dystrophy type 1A [58]. Metformin therapy promotes weight growth and energy efficiency, improves muscular function, and improves skeletal muscle histology in female dy2J/dy2J mice (but not in male dy2J/dy2J mice) [58]. Metformin also improved the mobility and walking abilities of people with myotonic dystrophy [59]. Metformin has also been shown to increase autophagy and provide cardioprotection in a mouse model deficient in δ-sarcoglycan, a protein encoded by the SGCD gene and associated with LGMD R6 (LGMD2F) [60].

2.7 Tranilast: From allergies to Duchenne cardiomyopathy

The life expectancy of DMD patients has improved recently due to advancements in the prevention of respiratory complications, however, there has been a notable increase in advanced cardiomyopathy symptoms [61]. To eventually cure DMD, gene replacement or other correction therapy must also approach the existence of fibrosis [62]. Furthermore, this concept favors DMD patients who develop DCM, marked by inflammation, fibrosis, and necrosis [63]. A compound with anti-fibrotic properties is *tranilast*, an anti-allergic agent and a calcium channel blocker prescribed for over 30 years to adults and children [64]. In mdx mice, improving muscle pathology and motor performance with Ca-handling drugs prevented aberrant intracellular Ca influx through the transient receptor potential cation channel, subfamily V 2 (TRPV2) [65]. The results of a single-arm, open-label, multicenter study on the safety and efficacy of tranilast for heart failure in patients with MDs—of whom the vast majority were DMD patients—were published in 2022 by Matsumura and colleagues [66]. Although there was no significant improvement in cardiac function, the authors concluded that tranilast was safe and effective in inhibiting TRPV2 expression and may represent a viable medication for patients with early heart failure [66].

Even in MD patients with advanced heart failure, tranilast is safe and effective at inhibiting TRPV2 expression.

2.8 Phosphodiesterase type 5 inhibitors

Increased muscle damage and irregular blood flow after muscle contraction—the condition known as functional ischemia—are hallmarks of DMD [67]. Thus, multiple pathways have been studied in the past decades to alleviate the ischemic picture in MDs. A potential novel therapeutic target for DMD is the nitric oxide (NO) - cyclic guanosine monophosphate (cGMP) pathway. *Phosphodiesterase type 5 (PDE5) inhibitors*, which extend the half-life of cGMP, have been shown to improve the function of the limb, respiratory, and cardiac muscles in mdx mice and to increase the lifespan of dystrophin-deficient zebrafish [68–70]. Since their major indication is erectile dysfunction, PDE5 can be considered as repurposed therapy in MDs. There are four major types of PDE5 inhibitors approved by the FDA [71] of which *sildenafil* and *tadalafil* were the most studied outside of their intended use. According to a 2012 study by Percival and colleagues, sildenafil administration for 14 weeks decreased diaphragm muscle weakness and supported normal extracellular matrix organization in mdx animals [72]. However, a placebo-controlled phase II trial (REVERSE DBMD; [73] including patients with Duchenne and Becker MD was terminated earlier due to worsening cardiomyopathy in some of the patients who received sildenafil [72]. As a PDE inhibitor tadalafil is more selective for PDE5 than sildenafil [74], which is why its evaluation advanced to a randomized, placebo-controlled phase III trial [73] that enrolled 331 patients. Nevertheless, tadalafil did not demonstrate efficacy in reducing the decline of walking ability in the treated group [75].

2.9 A new perspective on antibiotics

Since the early 1990s, it has been recognized that some antibiotics may reduce premature termination codons in eukaryotic cells [76]. In animal studies, the antibiotic family known as aminoglycosides has been shown to prevent nonsense mutations [24]. Thus, it was only a matter of time before researchers used this compound in

MDs. Barton-Davis and colleagues reported in 1999 that subcutaneous injections of gentamicin restored dystrophin levels in the skeletal muscles of mdx mice, demonstrating the potential of this family of antibiotics for the first time in *in vivo* [77].

Stretch-activated channels (SACs) are another pathway that has been proposed as being relevant in the pathophysiology of DMD [78]. These channels are permeable to Na^+ and Ca^2 and respond to mechanical stress [79, 80]. Lack of dystrophin increases skeletal muscle SAC activity in mdx mice [81–83]. Therefore, in muscles exhibiting various degrees of the dystrophic phenotype, researchers looked at the transient receptor potential canonical channel 1 (TRPC1) level and the effects of streptomycin, a SAC blocker [78]. In diaphragm and sternomastoid muscles, streptomycin decreased creatine kinase and reduced exercise-induced increases in total calcium and Evans blue dye absorption (a sensitive and early marker of myofiber injury) [78]. However, it must be taken into account when using aminoglycosides, that these drugs present various levels of oto- and/or nephrotoxicity [84, 85].

In 2003, the group led by Politano published the results of a small study on four patients with DMD. Immunohistochemistry and immunoblotting showed that dystrophin re-expression occurred in muscle biopsies performed after gentamicin treatment in three out of four patients that presented a more permissive UGA stop codon [86]. Seven years later, Malik and colleagues published the results of a multicenter trial that evaluated the safety of gentamicin infusions twice a week for 6 months [87]. Except for one patient who received an incorrectly calculated dosage, no patient showed a decreased renal or hearing function. The study's second goal was to see whether gentamicin improved muscular strength and increased dystrophin binding at the muscle membrane. Dystrophin levels significantly improved ($p = 0.027$) after 6 months of gentamicin treatment, and this was associated with a decrease in serum CK [88].

2.10 Tyrosine kinase inhibitors

Muscle degeneration and poor muscle regeneration brought on by a lack of dystrophin are major characteristics of DMD pathophysiology [89]. Several variables, including a reduction in satellite cell (SC) capacity (the critical precursors to myogenesis), have been linked to this defective regeneration [90]. SC proliferation and self-renewal in response to resistance training and muscle damage depend on the interleukin-6 (IL-6) cytokine's activation of the signal transducer and activator of transcription 3 (STAT3) [91–93]. Sunitinib is a multi-targeted tyrosine kinase inhibitor and a therapeutic option for treating renal cell carcinoma, gastrointestinal stromal tumors, and progressive, well-differentiated, advanced panNETs [24, 94]. Sunitinib was evaluated for its efficacy in the mdx mice model of DMD, in which it demonstrated the ability to induce muscle regeneration via transient STAT3 activation [90]. Furthermore, in 2022, Oliveira-Santos and colleagues published the results of an interesting study that evaluated how long-term sunitinib use affected heart pathology and function in mdx mouse model. The authors concluded that sunitinib increased cardiac electrical performance and reduced ventricular hypertrophy, cardiomyocyte membrane damage, and fibrotic tissue deposition in the heart muscle of mdx animals via lowered STAT3 phosphorylation [95].

Nintedanib is also a tyrosine kinase inhibitor approved for treating idiopathic pulmonary fibrosis (IPF) [96].

Previous studies on primary lung fibroblasts and dermal fibroblasts from patients with IPF and systemic sclerosis have demonstrated the anti-fibrotic activity of nintedanib, thus rendering this compound a potential aid in DMD [97, 98]. A one-month course of nintedanib therapy in mdx mice reduced skeletal muscle fibrosis and improved muscle function, thus reinforcing the idea that tyrosine kinase inhibitors could have a potential role for clinical exploration in DMD [99].

3. Conclusions

Recent scientific breakthroughs have enhanced diagnostic skills and permitted experimental research into gene therapy and standard pharmacological therapies, eventually leading to successful treatments for many inherited disorders.

Among them, muscular dystrophies and genetic diseases caused by mutations in over 40 genes result in dystrophic alterations on muscle biopsy and cause progressive weakness and degeneration of skeletal muscles. Due to advances in molecular biology techniques and an understanding of the mechanisms underlying these diseases, the genetic defect of most muscular dystrophies can now be precisely determined. Also, specialized therapy to help patients can be provided for some types of dystrophies, while many others are in the advanced clinical development stage. Although advances in the management and care of people with these disorders have slowed disease progression, more research is needed because the patients still face a lack of effective treatments. As a result, new forms of therapies are required. Repurposing existing intensively studied drugs with well-known pharmacokinetic, pharmacodynamic, tolerability, and safety profiles holds promise for timely effective therapies for patients suffering from life-threatening conditions who cannot wait for a traditional drug development cycle. Quickly redirecting these drugs to other directions can improve life expectancy and quality of life in affected patients. The use of this path is accelerated by incentives, guidance, and protection provided by holding an orphan drug designation status. Drug repurposing is a valuable strategy with enormous potential for delivering long-awaited therapies that may be safeguarded by orphan drug designation status, enabling successful, fair-priced commercialization.

Acknowledgements

This work was funded by the Ministry of Research, Innovation, and Digitalization in Romania, under Program 1—The Improvement of the National System of Research and Development, Subprogram 1.2—Institutional Excellence-Projects of Excellence Funding in RDI, Contract No. 31PFE/30.12.2021. National Program 31 N/2016/PN 16.22.02.05 and National Program 10 N/2023/PN 23.16.01.02.

Conflict of interest

The authors declare no conflict of interest.

Author details

Ioana Lambrescu[1,2], Emilia Manole[1,3], Laura Cristina Ceafalan[1,2] and Gisela Gaina[1*]

1 Cell Biology, Neurosciences and Experimental Myology Laboratory, Victor Babes Institute of Pathology, Bucharest, Romania

2 Department of Cellular and Molecular Biology and Histology, Carol Davila University of Medicine and Pharmacy, Bucharest, Romania

3 Pathology Department, Colentina Clinical Hospital, Bucharest, Romania

*Address all correspondence to: gisela.gaina@ivb.ro

IntechOpen

© 2023 The Author(s). Licensee IntechOpen. This chapter is distributed under the terms of the Creative Commons Attribution License (http://creativecommons.org/licenses/by/3.0), which permits unrestricted use, distribution, and reproduction in any medium, provided the original work is properly cited.

References

[1] Datta N, Ghosh PS. Update on muscular dystrophies with focus on novel treatments and biomarkers. Current Neurology and Neuroscience Reports [Internet]. 2020;**20**(6):14. Available from: https://link.springer.com/10.1007/s11910-020-01034-6

[2] Carter JC, Sheehan DW, Prochoroff A, Birnkrant DJ. Muscular dystrophies. Clinics in Chest Medicine [Internet]. 2018;**39**(2):377-389. Available from: https://linkinghub.elsevier.com/retrieve/pii/S0272523118300042

[3] Mercuri E, Bönnemann CG, Muntoni F. Muscular dystrophies. Lancet. 2019;**394**(10213):2025-2038. [Internet] Available from: https://linkinghub.elsevier.com/retrieve/pii/S0140673619329101

[4] Sahoo BM, BVV RK, Sruti J, Mahapatra MK, Banik BK, Borah P. Drug repurposing strategy (DRS): Emerging approach to identify potential therapeutics for treatment of novel coronavirus infection. Frontiers in Molecular Biosciences [Internet]. 2021;**8**:628144. Available from: https://www.frontiersin.org/articles/10.3389/fmolb.2021.628144/full

[5] Examination of clinical trial costs and barriers for drug development [Internet]. Available from: https://aspe.hhs.gov/sites/default/files/migrated_legacy_files//44516/rpt_erg.pdf

[6] Development & Approval Process | Drugs. Available from: www.fda.gov/Drugs/DevelopmentApprovalProcess

[7] Examination of clinical trial costs and barriers for drug development. Available from: https://aspe.hhs.gov/reports/examination-clinical-trial-costs-barriers-drug-development-0

[8] Andreana I, Repellin M, Carton F, Kryza D, Briançon S, Chazaud B, et al. Nanomedicine for gene delivery and drug repurposing in the treatment of muscular dystrophies. Pharmaceutics [Internet]. 2021;**13**(2):278. Available from: https://www.mdpi.com/1999-4923/13/2/278

[9] Koenig M, Hoffman EP, Bertelson CJ, Monaco AP, Feener C, Kunkel LM. Complete cloning of the duchenne muscular dystrophy (DMD) cDNA and preliminary genomic organization of the DMD gene in normal and affected individuals. Cell. [Internet]. 1987;**50**(3):509-517. Available from: https://linkinghub.elsevier.com/retrieve/pii/0092867487905046

[10] Ryder S, Leadley RM, Armstrong N, Westwood M, de Kock S, Butt T, et al. The burden, epidemiology, costs and treatment for Duchenne muscular dystrophy: An evidence review. Orphanet Journal of Rare Diseases [Internet]. 2017;**12**(1):79. Available from: http://ojrd.biomedcentral.com/articles/10.1186/s13023-017-0631-3

[11] Shieh PB. Emerging strategies in the treatment of Duchenne muscular dystrophy. Neurotherapeutics [Internet]. 2018;**15**(4):840-848. Available from: http://link.springer.com/10.1007/s13311-018-00687-z

[12] Ervasti JM, Ohlendieck K, Kahl SD, Gaver MG, Campbell KP. Deficiency of a glycoprotein component of the dystrophin complex in dystrophic muscle. Nature [Internet]. 1990;**345**(6273):315-319. Available from: http://www.nature.com/articles/345315a0

[13] Hoffman EP, Brown RH, Kunkel LM. Dystrophin: The protein product of the

duchenne muscular dystrophy locus. Cell [Internet]. 1987;**51**(6):919-928. Available from: https://linkinghub.elsevier.com/retrieve/pii/0092867487905794

[14]] McNally E. Novel targets and approaches to treating skeletal muscle disease. In: Muscle, Fundamental Biology and Mechanisms of Disease. Amsterdam, The Netherlands: Elsevier; 2012;**2**:1095-1103. Available from: https://linkinghub.elsevier.com/retrieve/pii/B9780123815101000818

[15] Wu R, Song Y, Wu S, Chen Y. Promising therapeutic approaches of utrophin replacing dystrophin in the treatment of Duchenne muscular dystrophy. Fundamental Research [Internet]. 2022;**2**(6):885-893. Available from: https://linkinghub.elsevier.com/retrieve/pii/S266732582200293X

[16] Skeletal muscle specific IRES activity of Utrophin A is enhanced by eEF1A2. Available from: https://central.bac-lac.gc.ca/.item?id=MR86675&op=pdf&app=Library&oclc_number=1019493836)

[17] Péladeau C, Adam N, Bronicki LM, Coriati A, Thabet M, Al-Rewashdy H, et al. Identification of therapeutics that target eEF1A2 and upregulate utrophin a translation in dystrophic muscles. Nature Communications. 2020;**11**(1):1990. [Internet] Available from: http://www.nature.com/articles/s41467-020-15971-w

[18] Disatnik M-H, Dhawan J, Yu Y, Beal MF, Whirl MM, Franco AA, et al. Evidence of oxidative stress in mdx mouse muscle: Studies of the pre-necrotic state. Journal of the Neurological Sciences [Internet]. 1998;**161**(1):77-84 Available from: https://linkinghub.elsevier.com/retrieve/pii/S0022510X98002585

[19] Irwin WA, Bergamin N, Sabatelli P, Reggiani C, Megighian A, Merlini L, et al. Mitochondrial dysfunction and apoptosis in myopathic mice with collagen VI deficiency. Nature Genetics. [Internet]. 2003;**35**(4):367-371. Available from: http://www.nature.com/articles/ng1270

[20] Terrill JR, Radley-Crabb HG, Iwasaki T, Lemckert FA, Arthur PG, Grounds MD. Oxidative stress and pathology in muscular dystrophies: Focus on protein thiol oxidation and dysferlinopathies. The FEBS Journal. [Internet]. 2013;**280**(17):4149-4164. Available from: https://onlinelibrary.wiley.com/doi/10.1111/febs.12142

[21] Menazza S, Blaauw B, Tiepolo T, Toniolo L, Braghetta P, Spolaore B, et al. Oxidative stress by monoamine oxidases is causally involved in myofiber damage in muscular dystrophy. Human Molecular Genetics [Internet]. 2010;**19**(21):4207-4215. Available from: https://academic.oup.com/hmg/article-lookup/doi/10.1093/hmg/ddq339

[22] Youdim MBH, Edmondson D, Tipton KF. The therapeutic potential of monoamine oxidase inhibitors. Nature Reviews. Neuroscience [Internet]. 2006;**7**(4):295-309. Available from: http://www.nature.com/articles/nrn1883

[23] Blair HA, Dhillon S. Safinamide: A review in Parkinson's disease. CNS Drugs [Internet]. 2017;**31**(2):169-176. Available from: http://link.springer.com/10.1007/s40263-017-0408-1

[24] Vitiello L, Marabita M, Sorato E, Nogara L, Forestan G, Mouly V, et al. Drug repurposing for Duchenne muscular dystrophy: The monoamine oxidase B inhibitor safinamide ameliorates the pathological phenotype in mdx mice and in myogenic cultures from DMD patients. Frontiers in Physiology [Internet]. 2018;**9**:1087. Available from: https://www.frontiersin.org/article/10.3389/fphys.2018.01087/full

[25] Dalmaz Y, Peyrin L, Mamelle JC, Tuil D, Gilly R, Cier JF. The pattern of urinary catecholamines and their metabolites in Duchenne myopathy, in relation to disease evolution. Journal of Neural Transmission. 1979;**46**(1):17-34. [Internet] Available from: http://link.springer.com/10.1007/BF01243426

[26] Jordan VC. Tamoxifen: A most unlikely pioneering medicine. Nature Reviews. Drug Discovery [Internet]. 2003;**2**(3):205-213. Available from: http://www.nature.com/articles/nrd1031

[27] Arnott J, Martinkovich S, Planey SL,Shah D. Selective estrogen receptor modulators: Tissue specificity and clinical utility. Clinical Interventions in Aging. 2014;**9**:1437-1452. Available from: http://www.dovepress.com/selective-estrogen-receptor-modulators-tissue-specificity-and-clinical-peer-reviewed-article-CIA

[28] Mahmoodzadeh S, Eder S, Nordmeyer J, Ehler E, Huber O, Martus P, et al. Estrogen receptor alpha up-regulation and redistribution in human heart failure. The FASEB Journal [Internet]. 2006;**20**(7):926-934. Available from: https://onlinelibrary.wiley.com/doi/10.1096/fj.05-5148com

[29] Koot RW, Amelink GJ, Blankenstein MA, Bär PR. Tamoxifen and oestrogen both protect the rat muscle against physiological damage. The Journal of Steroid Biochemistry and Molecular Biology. [Internet]. 1991;**40**(4-6):689-IN10. Available from: https://linkinghub.elsevier.com/retrieve/pii/096007609190292D

[30] Custódio JA, Dinis TCP, Almeida LM, Madeira VMC. Tamoxifen and hydroxytamoxifen as intramembraneous inhibitors of lipid peroxidation. Evidence for peroxyl radical scavenging activity. Biochemical Pharmacology [Internet]. 1994;**47**(11):1989-1998. Available from: https://linkinghub.elsevier.com/retrieve/pii/0006295294900736

[31] Dodds ML, Kargacin ME, Kargacin GJ. Effects of anti-oestrogens and β-estradiol on calcium uptake by cardiac sarcoplasmic reticulum. British Journal of Pharmacology [Internet]. 2001;**132**(7):1374-1382. Available from: http://doi.wiley.com/10.1038/sj.bjp.0703924

[32] Patel BM, Desai VJ. Beneficial role of tamoxifen in experimentally induced cardiac hypertrophy. Pharmacol Reports. 2014;**66**(2):264-272. [Internet] Available from: https://linkinghub.elsevier.com/retrieve/pii/S1734114014000449

[33] Dorchies OM, Reutenauer-Patte J, Dahmane E, Ismail HM, Petermann O, Patthey-Vuadens O, et al. The anticancer drug tamoxifen counteracts the pathology in a mouse model of Duchenne muscular dystrophy. The American Journal of Pathology. 2013;**182**(2):485-504. [Internet] Available from: https://linkinghub.elsevier.com/retrieve/pii/S0002944012008127

[34] Available from: https://www.duchenneuk.org/no-strong-evidence-for-tamoxifen-as-a-treatment-for-duchenne-muscular-dystrophy

[35] Bertorini TE, Palmieri GMA, Griffin J, Igarashi M, Hinton A, Karas JG. Effect of dantrolene in Duchenne muscular dystrophy. Muscle & Nerve. 1991;**14**(6):503-507. [Internet] Available from: https://onlinelibrary.wiley.com/doi/10.1002/mus.880140603

[36] Glahn KPE, Bendixen D, Girard T, Hopkins PM, Johannsen S, Rüffert H, et al. Availability of dantrolene for the management of malignant hyperthermia crises: European malignant hyperthermia group guidelines. British Journal of

Anaesthesia. 2020;**125**(2):133-140. [Internet] Available from: https://linkinghub.elsevier.com/retrieve/pii/S0007091220303494

[37] Kendall GC, Mokhonova EI, Moran M, Sejbuk NE, Wang DW, Silva O, et al. Dantrolene enhances antisense-mediated exon skipping in human and mouse models of Duchenne muscular dystrophy. Science Translational Medicine [Internet]. 2012;**4**(164):164ra160. Available from: https://www.science.org/doi/10.1126/scitranslmed.3005054

[38] Eser G, Topaloğlu H. Current outline of exon skipping trials in duchenne muscular dystrophy. Genes (Basel) [Internet]. 2022;**13**(7):1241. Available from: https://www.mdpi.com/2073-4425/13/7/1241

[39] Quinlan JG, Johnson SR, Samaha FJ. Letter to the editor. Muscle & Nerve. 1990;**13**(3):268-269. [Internet] Available from: https://onlinelibrary.wiley.com/doi/10.1002/mus.880130316

[40] Barthélémy F, Wang RT, Hsu C, Douine ED, Marcantonio EE, Nelson SF, et al. Targeting RyR activity boosts antisense exon 44 and 45 skipping in human DMD skeletal or cardiac muscle culture models. Molecular Therapy - Nucleic Acids [Internet]. 2019;**18**:580-589. Available from: https://linkinghub.elsevier.com/retrieve/pii/S2162253119302677

[41] Sanders SP. Did they lower stress in the trial? Journal of the American College of Cardiology [Internet]. 2005;**45**(6):858-859. Available from: https://linkinghub.elsevier.com/retrieve/pii/S0735109704024994

[42] Matsumura T. Beta-blockers in children with Duchenne cardiomyopathy. Reviews on Recent Clinical Trials. 2014;**9**(2):76-81. [Internet] Available from: http://www.eurekaselect.com/openurl/content.php?genre=article&issn=1574-8871&volume=9&issue=2&spage=76

[43] Mallouk N, Jacquemond V, Allard B. Elevated subsarcolemmal Ca 2+ in mdx mouse skeletal muscle fibers detected with Ca 2+ –activated K + channels. Proceedings of the National Academy of Sciences [Internet]. 2000;**97**(9):4950-4955. Available from: https://pnas.org/doi/full/10.1073/pnas.97.9.4950

[44] Phillips MF, Quinlivan R. Calcium antagonists for Duchenne muscular dystrophy. Cochrane Database of Systematic Reviews [Internet]. 2008;**8**(4):CD004571. Available from: https://doi.wiley.com/10.1002/14651858.CD004571.pub2

[45] Emery A. Verapamil in Duchenne muscular dystrophy. Lancet [Internet]. 1982;**319**(8271):559. Available from: https://linkinghub.elsevier.com/retrieve/pii/S0140673682920633

[46] Matsumura CY, Pertille A, Albuquerque TCP, Santo Neto H, Marques MJ. Diltiazem and verapamil protect dystrophin-deficient muscle fibers of MDX mice from degeneration: A potential role in calcium buffering and sarcolemmal stability. Muscle & Nerve. 2009;**39**(2):167-176. [Internet] Available from: https://onlinelibrary.wiley.com/doi/10.1002/mus.21188

[47] Altamirano F, Valladares D, Henríquez-Olguín C, Casas M, López JR, Allen PD, et al. Nifedipine treatment reduces resting calcium concentration, oxidative and apoptotic gene expression, and improves muscle function in dystrophic MDX mice. PLoS One [Internet]. 2013;**8**(12):e81222. Available from: https://dx.plos.org/10.1371/journal.pone.0081222

[48] Inzucchi SE, Bergenstal RM, Buse JB, Diamant M, Ferrannini E, Nauck M,

et al. Management of hyperglycemia in type 2 diabetes, 2015: A patient-centered approach: Update to a position statement of the American Diabetes Association and the European Association for the Study of diabetes. Diabetes Care. 2015;**38**(1):140-149. Available from: https://diabetesjournals.org/care/article/38/1/140/37869/Management-of-Hyperglycemia-in-Type-2-Diabetes

[49] Rotermund C, Machetanz G, Fitzgerald JC. The therapeutic potential of metformin in neurodegenerative diseases. Front Endocrinol (Lausanne) [Internet]. 2018;**9**:400. Available from: https://www.frontiersin.org/article/10.3389/fendo.2018.00400/full

[50] Ursini F, Russo E, Pellino G, D'Angelo S, Chiaravalloti A, De Sarro G, et al. Metformin and autoimmunity: A "new Deal" of an old drug. Frontiers in Immunology. 2018;**9**:1236. Available from: https://www.frontiersin.org/article/10.3389/fimmu.2018.01236/full

[51] Pernicova I, Korbonits M. Metformin—Mode of action and clinical implications for diabetes and cancer. Nature Reviews. Endocrinology [Internet]. 2014;**10**(3):143-156. Available from: http://www.nature.com/articles/nrendo.2013.256

[52] García-Puga M, Saenz-Antoñanzas A, Matheu A, López de Munain A. Targeting myotonic dystrophy type 1 with metformin. International Journal of Molecular Sciences [Internet]. 2022;**23**(5):2901. Available from: https://www.mdpi.com/1422-0067/23/5/2901

[53] Mantuano P, Sanarica F, Conte E, Morgese MG, Capogrosso RF, Cozzoli A, et al. Effect of a long-term treatment with metformin in dystrophic mdx mice: A reconsideration of its potential clinical interest in Duchenne muscular dystrophy. Biochemical Pharmacology. 2018;**154**:89-103. [Internet] Available from: https://linkinghub.elsevier.com/retrieve/pii/S0006295218301655

[54] Chen J, Lai X. C–X–C motif chemokine ligand 12: A potential therapeutic target in Duchenne muscular dystrophy. Bioengineered. 2021;**12**(1):5428-5439. Available from: https://www.tandfonline.com/doi/full/10.1080/21655979.2021.1967029

[55] Lin C, Han G, Jia L, Zhao Y, Song J, Ran N, et al. Cardio-respiratory and phenotypic rescue of dystrophin/utrophin-deficient mice by combination therapy. EMBO Reports. 2022;**23**(6):e53955. [Internet] Available from: https://onlinelibrary.wiley.com/doi/10.15252/embr.202153955

[56] Casteels K, Fieuws S, van Helvoirt M, Verpoorten C, Goemans N, Coudyzer W, et al. Metformin therapy to reduce weight gain and visceral adiposity in children and adolescents with neurogenic or myogenic motor deficit. Pediatric Diabetes. 2010;**11**(1):61-69. [Internet] Available from: https://onlinelibrary.wiley.com/doi/10.1111/j.1399-5448.2009.00512.x

[57] Clinical trial. Available from: 10.1001/jamanetworkopen.2019.14171

[58] Fontes-Oliveira CC, Oliveira MBS, Körner Z, Harandi VM, Durbeej M. Effects of metformin on congenital muscular dystrophy type 1A disease progression in mice: A gender impact study. Scientific Reports. [Internet]. 2018;**8**(1):16302. Available from: http://www.nature.com/articles/s41598-018-34362-2

[59] Bassez G, Audureau E, Hogrel J-Y, Arrouasse R, Baghdoyan S, Bhugaloo H, et al. Improved mobility with metformin in patients with myotonic dystrophy type 1: A randomized controlled trial. Brain [Internet]. 2018;**141**(10):2855-2865 Available from: https://academic.oup.com/brain/article/141/10/2855/5086409

[60] Kanamori H, Naruse G, Yoshida A, Minatoguchi S, Watanabe T, Kawaguchi T, et al. Metformin enhances autophagy and provides cardioprotection in δ-sarcoglycan deficiency-induced dilated cardiomyopathy. Circulation Heart failure. 2019;**12**(4):e005418. Available from: https://www.ahajournals.org/doi/10.1161/CIRCHEARTFAILURE.118.005418

[61] Adorisio R, Mencarelli E, Cantarutti N, Grandinetti M. Cardiomyopathy in Duchenne muscular distrophy: Clinical insights and therapeutic implications. In: Cardiomyopathy - Disease of the Heart Muscle. London, UK, London: IntechOpen; 2021. Available from: https://www.intechopen.com/books/cardiomyopathy-disease-of-the-heart-muscle/cardiomyopathy-in-duchenne-muscular-distrophy-clinical-insights-and-therapeutic-implications

[62] Muir LA, Chamberlain JS. Emerging strategies for cell and gene therapy of the muscular dystrophies. Expert Reviews in Molecular Medicine. 2009;**11**:e18. [Internet] Available from: https://www.cambridge.org/core/product/identifier/S1462399409001100/type/journal_article

[63] Farini A, Gowran A, Bella P, Sitzia C, Scopece A, Castiglioni E, et al. Fibrosis rescue improves cardiac function in dystrophin-deficient mice and Duchenne patient–specific cardiomyocytes by immunoproteasome modulation. The American Journal of Pathology. 2019;**189**(2):339-353. [Internet] Available from: https://linkinghub.elsevier.com/retrieve/pii/S0002944018303705

[64] Matsumura T, Hashimoto H, Sekimizu M, Saito AM, Iwata Y, Asakura M, et al. Study protocol for a multicenter, open-label, single-arm study of tranilast for cardiomyopathy of muscular dystrophy. The Kurume Medical Journal [Internet]. 2019;**66**(2):MS662006. Available from: https://www.jstage.jst.go.jp/article/kurumemedj/66/2/66_MS662006/_article

[65] Iwata Y, Katanosaka Y, Shijun Z, Kobayashi Y, Hanada H, Shigekawa M, et al. Protective effects of Ca2+ handling drugs against abnormal Ca2+ homeostasis and cell damage in myopathic skeletal muscle cells. Biochemical Pharmacology. 2005;**70**(5):740-751. [Internet] Available from: https://linkinghub.elsevier.com/retrieve/pii/S0006295205003655

[66] Matsumura T, Hashimoto H, Sekimizu M, Saito AM, Motoyoshi Y, Nakamura A, et al. Tranilast for advanced heart failure in patients with muscular dystrophy: A single-arm, open-label, multicenter study. Orphanet Journal of Rare Diseases [Internet]. 2022;**17**(1):201. Available from: https://ojrd.biomedcentral.com/articles/10.1186/s13023-022-02352-3

[67] Asai A, Sahani N, Kaneki M, Ouchi Y, Martyn JAJ, Yasuhara SE. Primary role of functional ischemia, quantitative evidence for the two-hit mechanism, and phosphodiesterase-5 inhibitor therapy in mouse muscular dystrophy. PLoS One [Internet]. 2007;**2**(8):e806. Available from: https://dx.plos.org/10.1371/journal.pone.0000806

[68] Kobayashi YM, Rader EP, Crawford RW, Iyengar NK, Thedens DR, Faulkner JA, et al. Sarcolemma-localized nNOS is required to maintain activity after mild exercise. Nature [Internet]. 2008;**456**(7221):511-515. Available from: http://www.nature.com/articles/nature07414

[69] Thomas GD, Ye J, De Nardi C, Monopoli A, Ongini E, Victor RG. Treatment with a nitric oxide-donating NSAID alleviates functional muscle ischemia in the mouse model of Duchenne muscular dystrophy. PLoS One

[Internet]. 2012;**7**(11):e49350. Available from: https://dx.plos.org/10.1371/journal.pone.0049350

[70] Kawahara G, Karpf JA, Myers JA, Alexander MS, Guyon JR, Kunkel LM. Drug screening in a zebrafish model of Duchenne muscular dystrophy. Proceedings of the National Academy of Sciences [Internet]. 2011;**108**(13):5331-5336. Available from: https://pnas.org/doi/full/10.1073/pnas.1102116108

[71] Ahmed WS, Geethakumari AM, Biswas KH. Phosphodiesterase 5 (PDE5): Structure-function regulation and therapeutic applications of inhibitors. Biomedicine & Pharmacotherapy. 2021;**134**:111128. [Internet] Available from: https://linkinghub.elsevier.com/retrieve/pii/S0753332220313214

[72] Percival JM, Whitehead NP, Adams ME, Adamo CM, Beavo JA, Froehner SC. Sildenafil reduces respiratory muscle weakness and fibrosis in the mdx mouse model of Duchenne muscular dystrophy. The Journal of Pathology [Internet]. 2012;**228**(1):77-87. Available from: https://onlinelibrary.wiley.com/doi/10.1002/path.4054

[73] Available from: https://clinicaltrials.gov/ct2/show/NCT01462292

[74] Wright PJ. Comparison of phosphodiesterase type 5 (PDE5) inhibitors. International Journal of Clinical Practice [Internet]. 2006;**60**(8):967-975. Available from: https://onlinelibrary.wiley.com/doi/10.1111/j.1742-1241.2006.01049.x

[75] Victor RG, Sweeney HL, Finkel R, McDonald CM, Byrne B, Eagle M, et al. A phase 3 randomized placebo-controlled trial of tadalafil for Duchenne muscular dystrophy. Neurology [Internet]. 2017;**89**(17):1811-1820. Available from: https://www.neurology.org/lookup/doi/10.1212/WNL.0000000000004570

[76] Bertoni C, Namgoong J. Clinical potential of ataluren in the treatment of Duchenne muscular dystrophy. Degenerative Neurological and Neuromuscular Disease. 2016;**37**:37-48. Available from: https://www.dovepress.com/clinical-potential-of-ataluren-in-the-treatment-of-duchenne-muscular-d-peer-reviewed-article-DNND

[77] Barton-Davis ER, Cordier L, Shoturma DI, Leland SE, Sweeney HL. Aminoglycoside antibiotics restore dystrophin function to skeletal muscles of mdx mice. The Journal of Clinical Investigation [Internet]. 1999;**104**(4):375-381. Available from: http://www.jci.org/articles/view/7866

[78] Matsumura CY, Taniguti APT, Pertille A, Neto HS, Marques MJ. Stretch-activated calcium channel protein TRPC1 is correlated with the different degrees of the dystrophic phenotype in mdx mice. American Journal of Physiology. Cell Physiology [Internet]. 2011;**301**(6):C1344-C1350. Available from: https://www.physiology.org/doi/10.1152/ajpcell.00056.2011

[79] Franco A, Lansman JB. Calcium entry through stretch-inactivated ion channels in mdx myotubes. Nature [Internet]. 1990;**344**(6267):670-673. Available from: http://www.nature.com/articles/344670a0

[80] Franco A, Lansman JB. Stretch-sensitive channels in developing muscle cells from a mouse cell line. The Journal of Physiology [Internet]. 1990;**427**(1):361-380. Available from: https://onlinelibrary.wiley.com/doi/10.1113/jphysiol.1990.sp018176

[81] Franco-Obregón A, Lansman JB. Mechanosensitive ion channels in skeletal muscle from normal and dystrophic mice. The Journal of Physiology [Internet]. 1994;**481**(2):299-309.

Available from: https://onlinelibrary.wiley.com/doi/10.1113/jphysiol.1994.sp020440

[82] Yeung EW, Allen DG. Stretch-activated channels in stretch-induced muscle damage: Role in muscular dystrophy. Clinical and Experimental Pharmacology & Physiology. 2004;**31**(8):551-556. [Internet] Available from: https://onlinelibrary.wiley.com/doi/10.1111/j.1440-1681.2004.04027.x

[83] Vandebrouck C, Duport G, Cognard C, Raymond G. Cationic channels in normal and dystrophic human myotubes. Neuromuscular Disorders. 2001;**11**(1):72-79. [Internet] Available from: https://linkinghub.elsevier.com/retrieve/pii/S096089660000153X

[84] Forge A, Schacht J. Aminoglycoside Antibiotics. Audiology and Neurotology. 2000;**5**(1):3-22. [Internet] Available from: https://www.karger.com/Article/FullText/13861

[85] Mingeot-Leclercq M-P, Tulkens PM. Aminoglycosides: Nephrotoxicity. Antimicrobial Agents and Chemotherapy. 1999;**43**(5):1003-1012. [Internet] Available from: https://journals.asm.org/doi/10.1128/AAC.43.5.1003

[86] Politano L, Nigro G, Nigro V, Piluso G, Papparella S, Paciello O, et al. Gentamicin administration in Duchenne patients with premature stop codon. Preliminary results. Acta Myologica : Myopathies and Cardiomyopathies : Official Journal of the Mediterranean Society of Myology. 2003;**22**(1):15-21. [Internet] Available from: http://www.ncbi.nlm.nih.gov/pubmed/12966700

[87] Six month study of gentamicin in duchenne muscular dystrophy with stop codons. Available from: https://clinicaltrials.gov/ct2/show/NCT00451074

[88] Malik V, Rodino-Klapac LR, Viollet L, Wall C, King W, Al-Dahhak R, et al. Gentamicin-induced read through of stop codons in Duchenne muscular dystrophy. Annals of Neurology. 2010;**67**(6):771-780. NA-NA Available from: https://onlinelibrary.wiley.com/doi/10.1002/ana.22024

[89] Goldstein JA, McNally EM. Mechanisms of muscle weakness in muscular dystrophy. The Journal of General Physiology. 2010;**136**(1):29-34. [Internet] Available from: https://rupress.org/jgp/article/136/1/29/53227/Mechanisms-of-muscle-weakness-in-muscular

[90] Fontelonga TM, Jordan B, Nunes AM, Barraza-Flores P, Bolden N, Wuebbles RD, et al. Sunitinib promotes myogenic regeneration and mitigates disease progression in the mdx mouse model of Duchenne muscular dystrophy. Human Molecular Genetics. 2019;**28**(13):2120-2132. [Internet] Available from: https://academic.oup.com/hmg/article/28/13/2120/5365303

[91] Serrano AL, Baeza-Raja B, Perdiguero E, Jardí M, Muñoz-Cánoves P. Interleukin-6 is an essential regulator of satellite cell-mediated skeletal muscle hypertrophy. Cell Metabolism. 2008;**7**(1):33-44. [Internet] Available from: https://linkinghub.elsevier.com/retrieve/pii/S155041310700366X

[92] Begue G, Douillard A, Galbes O, Rossano B, Vernus B, Candau R, et al. Early activation of rat skeletal muscle IL-6/STAT1/STAT3 dependent gene expression in resistance exercise linked to hypertrophy. PLoS One [Internet]. 2013;**8**(2):e57141. Available from: https://dx.plos.org/10.1371/journal.pone.0057141

[93] Zhu H, Xiao F, Wang G, Wei X, Jiang L, Chen Y, et al. STAT3

regulates self-renewal of adult muscle satellite cells during injury-induced muscle regeneration. Cell Reports. 2016;**16**(8):2102-2115. [Internet] Available from: https://linkinghub.elsevier.com/retrieve/pii/S2211124716309597

[94] Vivanet G, Gervaso L, Laffi A, Rubino M, Spada F, Fazio N. Ten years-experience of sunitinib in the treatment of advanced pan-NETs: An update on safety profile. Expert Opinion on Drug Safety [Internet]. 2022;**21**(3):303-310. Available from: https://www.tandfonline.com/doi/full/10.1080/14740338.2022.2000964

[95] Oliveira-Santos A, Dagda M, Burkin DJ. Sunitinib inhibits STAT3 phosphorylation in cardiac muscle and prevents cardiomyopathy in the mdx mouse model of Duchenne muscular dystrophy. Human Molecular Genetics. 2022;**31**(14):2358-2369. [Internet] Available from: https://academic.oup.com/hmg/article/31/14/2358/6528270

[96] Highlights of prescribing information. Available from: https://www.accessdata.fda.gov/drugsatfda_docs/label/2014/205832s000lbl.pdf

[97] Huang J, Beyer C, Palumbo-Zerr K, Zhang Y, Ramming A, Distler A, et al. Nintedanib inhibits fibroblast activation and ameliorates fibrosis in preclinical models of systemic sclerosis. Annals of the Rheumatic Diseases. 2016;**75**(5):883-890. [Internet] Available from: https://ard.bmj.com/lookup/doi/10.1136/annrheumdis-2014-207109

[98] Hostettler KE, Zhong J, Papakonstantinou E, Karakiulakis G, Tamm M, Seidel P, et al. Anti-fibrotic effects of nintedanib in lung fibroblasts derived from patients with idiopathic pulmonary fibrosis. Respiratory Research [Internet]. 2014;**15**(1):157. Available from: https://respiratory-research.biomedcentral.com/articles/10.1186/s12931-014-0157-3

[99] Piñol-Jurado P, Suárez-Calvet X, Fernández-Simón E, Gallardo E, de la Oliva N, Martínez-Muriana A, et al. Nintedanib decreases muscle fibrosis and improves muscle function in a murine model of dystrophinopathy. Cell Death & Disease. 2018;**9**(7):776. [Internet] Available from: http://www.nature.com/articles/s41419-018-0792-6

Chapter 5

Advanced Physiotherapy Intervention for Muscular Dystrophy

Saina Swathi, Kandhili Chandrasekaran Gayathri and Purushothaman Senthil

Abstract

Muscular dystrophies are rare neuromuscular conditions which are genetically and clinically diverse that cause gradual, progressive weakness and breakdown of skeletal muscles over time. Gene mutations, typically in those involved in producing muscle proteins, are the primary cause of muscular dystrophy. Based on these gene mutations and proteins involved a wide variety of muscular dystrophies have been identified. The primary muscles affected, the level of weakness, the rate at which symptoms increase, and the onset of symptoms vary among different muscular dystrophies. Some forms are linked to issues with other organ systems. The kind of muscular dystrophy will be ascertained through a physical examination, medical history, and other diagnostic techniques. Currently, there is no cure for muscular dystrophy. Multidisciplinary management plays a vital role in increasing life expectancy and improving the quality of life. Physical therapy as a part of supportive care management can help muscular dystrophy patients in various ways. It can help in maintaining joint range of motion, flexibility, and overall fitness. It helps in maintaining muscle strength, improving range of motion, and reducing pain. In this chapter, we will present the advanced physiotherapeutic interventions helpful for subjects with muscular dystrophies, based on the evidence available in the literature.

Keywords: muscular dystrophy, physiotherapy, muscle strength, assistive devices, fall prevention

1. Introduction

Muscular dystrophies are inherited myogenic conditions distinguished by gradual muscle atrophy, variable distribution, and extreme weakness. Depending on the kind of muscular dystrophy, particular signs and symptoms appear at various ages and in various muscle groups. In muscular dystrophy, gene mutations prevent the body from making the necessary proteins for building healthy muscle [1]. According to estimates, there are 3.6 cases of muscular dystrophy per 100,000 persons worldwide. While the prevalence of the most prevalent types of muscular dystrophies, such as Duchene's and Beckers, is estimated to be 4.6 and 1.6 per 100,000 individuals, respectively, with Americans having the highest prevalence at 5.1 per 100,000 and Africans having the lowest prevalence at 1.7 per 100,000 people [2].

Studies evaluating the burden of care and utilization of resources in patients with degenerative myopathy were more prevalent in both newly diagnosed patients and those who already had the disease. Duchene's muscular dystrophy (MD) has a direct annual medical expenditure that can be anywhere between $20,000 and over $50,000. Medical expenses cover direct myopathy-related expenses and secondary issues such as cardiac, pulmonary, nutritional, and spine concerns. MD-related medical expenses rise along with their associated problems throughout time [3].

From the past centuries, the primary pattern of muscle involvement, age of onset, and other clinical characteristics have been used to categorise muscular dystrophies. Based on inheritance and the underlying genetic abnormality, subtypes were identified. Congenital muscular dystrophies typically manifest symptoms within the first few months of life or soon after birth. DMD and many limb-girdle muscular dystrophies appear in early infancy or adolescence, frequently after the development of independent ambulation. Myotonic dystrophy, facioscapulohumeral muscular dystrophy, and other limb-girdle muscular dystrophies typically present in adulthood [4].

An integrated approach that combines clinical signs, age of onset, distribution of muscle weakness, and cardiac involvement with specific diagnostic procedures like laboratory tests, muscle biopsy, muscle imaging, genetic testing, and brain imaging can help make a diagnosis of muscular dystrophies [5].

Pharmacological therapies used in the management and treatment of epilepsy, muscle tone, pain, and inflammation include anti-arrhythmic, anti-epileptic, anti-myotonic, non-steroidal anti-inflammatory medications (NSAIDs), and steroids. In order to achieve ambulation, surgical procedures including contracture release and spinal adjustments are useful. Muscular dystrophies can be prevented and managed with the use of genetic counselling, which should be given to the mother, female siblings, children, and any maternal relatives.

General supportive care, such as physical therapy, range-of-motion exercises, cushioning, skincare, orthotics, and safety awareness may be helpful in addition to pharmacological treatments [6].

2. Classification

According to their inheritance, age of onset, rate of progression, the extent and distribution of muscle weakness, and other related clinical symptoms, muscular dystrophies are divided into different categories.

2.1 Congenital muscular dystrophy (CMD)

A collection of autosomal recessive muscular dystrophies that either manifest at birth or before age. This group of dystrophies is categorised based on their phenotypic features into collagenopathies, merosinopathies, and Dystroglycanopathies. The primary clinical signs of the CMDs are hypotonia and progressive skeletal muscle weakening. These conditions may appear in diverse combinations of pulmonary, ophthalmologic, neurologic, gastrointestinal, cardiovascular, and neurologic symptoms [7]

2.2 Dystrophinopathies

Dystrophinopathies are of two forms, Severe one as Duchenne Muscular Dystrophy (DMD) phenotype and milder Beckers Muscular Dystrophy (BMD) phenotype.

2.2.1 Duchenne muscular dystrophy (DMD) phenotype

A most common form of muscular dystrophy with childhood and young onset. This X-Linked recessive disorder primarily affects male births and females are carriers. it is caused due to mutations in the DMD gene, which incorporates a protein called dystrophin. Its absence causes myofiber necrosis as well as progressive muscle weakness and fatigue. Progressive muscle weakness and wastage in the proximal lower limbs and trunk muscles, followed by upper limb and distal muscles. Delay in gross motor development, Gait abnormalities such as toe walking, and waddling gait. Difficulty in climbing the stairs, raising from the floor (Positive Gowers sign), and frequent falls. Secondary skeletal abnormalities such as reduction in bone density, risk of fractures, joint contractures, and Scoliosis. Respiratory symptoms such as ventilatory insufficiency, decreased cough capacity, respiratory tract infections, and sleep disorder breathing caused by Obstructive sleep apnea. Congestive heart failure, cardiac insufficiency, abnormal cardiac conduction, ventricular or supraventricular arrhythmias, and risk of unexpected early death are all consequences of progressive dilated cardiomyopathy. There are certain other symptoms like Cognitive decline, neuropsychological issues, and atypical neurobehavioral actions. Children with Duchenne MD now live longer and enjoy a much better quality of life due to advancements in multidisciplinary care. Many people live through their 30s, and some even into their 40s [8].

2.2.2 Beckers muscular dystrophy (BMD) phenotype

This kind of dystrophy is less severe than Duchenne muscular dystrophy. It can also be brought on by mutations in the dystrophin gene, which cause the muscles to have abnormally high or low quantities of the dystrophin protein. Compared to Duchenne, the symptoms do not manifest until later [9].

2.3 Emery-Dreyfuss muscular dystrophy (EDMD)

It is a relatively rare form of muscular dystrophy that falls into one of three inheritance categories: X-linked, autosomal dominant, or autosomal recessive. The pathogenesis of EDMD has been linked to a number of genes. To particular EDMD subtypes, EMD, LMNA, SYNE1, SYNE2, FHL1, and TMEM43 have all been identified. The four defining symptoms of EDMD are muscle weakness, early contractures, abnormal cardiac conduction, and cardiomyopathy, however, the presence and severity of these manifestations differ by subtype and person [10].

2.4 Limb-girdle muscular dystrophies (LGMD)

These conditions have been found to be a diverse set of myopathies that can affect people of all ages, from children to adults and range in severity. Depending on the mode of inheritance, the LGMDs are divided into two main groups: LGMD1 (autosomal dominant) and LGMD2 (autosomal recessive) [11]. The proximal muscles of the arms and legs are most significantly impacted by limb-girdle Dystrophies. Sometimes other patterns also include scapula peroneal, humeroperoneal and distal patterns of weakness. Associated issues with this kind of muscular dystrophy are cardiac involvement, Dysphagia, pulmonary complications and musculoskeletal spinal deformities [12].

2.5 Facioscapulohumeral dystrophy (FSHD)

Facioscapulohumeral dystrophy is the third most prevalent type of muscular dystrophy. This condition is of autosomal dominant inheritance. From early infancy through late adulthood, FSHD can start at any age. Although the deltoids are not affected, facial, periscapular, and humeral muscles are frequently affected early in the disease progression. FSHD usually advances slowly yet unevenly. Respiratory insufficiency and cardiac complications are rare when compared with retinal vascular diseases and hearing loss. Most patients with childhood onset have significant hearing loss which may impair language development [7].

2.6 Myotonic dystrophy (DM)

There are two different forms of myotonic muscular dystrophies, known as DM1 and DM2, which are autosomal dominant diseases characterised by increasing weakening, myotonia, and early-onset cataracts. A repeat expansion that removes or separates RNA-binding proteins and leads to improperly controlled alternative splicing is the root cause of both DM1 and DM2. The various symptoms linked to both disorders are most likely caused by the widespread dysregulation of alternative splicing. DM1 causes distal weakness in the long finger flexors, facial muscles, and ankle dorsiflexion. Myotonia (delayed muscle relaxation) is simpler to provoke in DM1 than in DM2 both clinically and electrodiagnostically. Proximal weakness and noticeable muscle discomfort are more prevalent in those with DM2. Despite these differences, these conditions can result in multisystem symptoms in the heart, gastrointestinal tract, and brain [13].

2.7 Oculopharyngeal dystrophy (OPMD)

Oculopharyngeal muscular dystrophy (OPMD), a late-onset myopathy, is defined by progressive ptosis, dysphagia, and proximal limb weakening. The polyadenine (poly[A]) binding protein nuclear 1 gene's exon 1 contains an aberrant extension of the alanine-encoding (GCN)n trinucleotide repeat, which is the source of the condition. Patients with OPMD may exhibit extra muscular symptoms like loss of respiratory function, particularly decreased forced expiratory volume, even while cardiac functions may still be intact. There have been instances of cohabitation with peripheral neuropathy, executive function problems, or dementia. The majority of the patients had problems walking and engaging in social activities, and nearly half of them reported feeling exhausted and in pain [14].

3. Management

The type of muscular dystrophy and its severity play a huge role in how an individual is managed. It comprises appropriate clinical oversight and symptomatic care. The therapy of individuals with muscular dystrophy requires a multidisciplinary team since they often exhibit a variety of clinical symptoms, including musculoskeletal, neurological, cardiovascular, pulmonary, and gastrointestinal issues. The medical expert who organises clinical treatment should actively involve the patient and their family in the process.

4. Advanced physiotherapy intervention for muscular dystrophy

Supportive physiotherapy is one of the strategies used to delay contractures and extend ambulation. It also plays an important role in the rehabilitation management of individuals with muscular dystrophy as these individuals are associated with several clinical manifestations depending upon the type of muscular dystrophy, they are suffering such as Musculo skeletal weakness, respiratory insufficiency, cardiac complications, gastrointestinal manifestations. This intervention's major objective is to keep unaffected muscle groups functioning as long as possible. Although exercise helps maintain muscle function, it can also increase the breakdown of muscle fibres. Depending on the severity of the condition, a customized exercise routine combined with advice from the rehabilitation team may enable them to live longer, more actively and independently thus improving their quality of life [15].

Stages of progression of Muscular dystrophy can be categorised simply into ambulatory and non-ambulatory stages. The further categorisation may also include pre-symptomatic, early and late ambulatory stages and early and late non-ambulatory stages.

In the early ambulatory and presymptomatic stages, Education, prevention strategies to keep muscles extensible, and contracture minimization. encouragement of proper activity and exercise. The provision of adaptable devices is crucial in supporting participation and function. when ambulatory and non-ambulatory stages are late. To enable maximum independence in everyday activities, function, and participation, it is helpful to provide an adequate wheelchair and seating as well as use assistive equipment and adaptations [16].

4.1 Muscle extensibility and joint mobility training

Due to abnormal muscle function, which results in restricted joint movement, muscle imbalance, prolonged static positioning, muscle imbalance, and fibrotic alterations in the muscle, people with muscular dystrophy have decreased muscle extensibility and joint contractures. The mobility of the chest wall is also impacted by this type of alteration, which causes breathing issues. Regular stretching of the ankle, knee, and hip should begin soon after a diagnosis and continue until adulthood.

Stretching of the upper extremities is essential in non-ambulatory stages. Under the supervision of physical and occupational therapists, a daily preventative home stretching plan should be initiated before the loss of passive ranges of motion.

Active stretching, active-assisted stretching, passive stretching, and long-term stretching using positioning, splinting, orthoses, and standing devices are all necessary for effective stretching of the musculotendinous unit. Standing programmes are advised as standing and walking become more challenging. Along with stretching techniques in order to prevent joint contractures use of manual therapy techniques, splinting, orthotic interventions, and serial casting are needed [17, 18]

4.2 Muscle strength and conditioning

Most of the muscular dystrophy subjects will have reduced muscle activity and increased fatigue as the disease progress gradually [12, 19].

For people with muscular dystrophy who are in the early ambulatory to early non-ambulatory stages of the disease, physiotherapists may advise gentle low-impact aerobic exercises that improve cardiovascular performance, increase muscle efficiency, and lessen fatigue. They may also advise aerobic exercises combined with supervised sub-maximal strength training programmes. If it is deemed medically safe, it may occasionally be extended until the late non-ambulatory periods. Supra-maximal and high-intensity exercises should be avoided because of the modest risk of exercise-induced muscle damage, myoglobinuria, and later overwork weakness due to the muscle degradation associated with muscular dystrophy.

Aerobic activities with a sub-maximal intensity of 60%–80% of the Target heart rate for 4 days/week can be trained. Mostly stationary bicycling and swimming and arm ergometers are preferable to treadmills. Strength training at a low intensity of less than 50% of individual 1 repetition Maximum and 10 repetitions each set with 3–5 sessions per day. Gradually increase the percentage of 1RM as tolerated over a period of weeks to months. Ensure that an adequate resting period between each session for 2–3 days is advisable to decrease the metabolic damage in muscular dystrophy.

The symptoms of exhaustion and myoglobinuria, which include feeling weaker rather than stronger 30 min after exercise, excessive muscle soreness 24–48 h later, severe muscle cramping, heaviness in the limbs, and significant shortness of breath, should be explained as muscular dystrophy patients participating in an exercise programme.

4.3 Fall prevention strategies

Muscular dystrophy subjects are more prone to falls due to the factors like muscle weakness, muscle imbalances, gait abnormalities and improper balance. Most of the falls occurring in the ambulatory stages are due to extrinsic factors such as slippery floors and objects on the floor acting as obstacles during ambulation.

In order to avoid falling the use of assistive and adaptive devices, such as orthoses, braces, canes, walkers, and hand splints, as well as home and environmental modifications are required. Sedentary behaviour should be minimised [20].

Possible modifications at home such as removing obstacles (toys, rugs, cords etc), and resting in a chair for home tasks instead of standing for prolonged periods help in fatigue management. Providing a handrail for stair climbing is needed. Learning Safe transfer techniques while using wheelchairs and other mobility devices under the supervision of the therapists. Floor modifications in the home by using non-slippery mats, non-slip treads for steps, Adaptive equipment for bathing, and Assistance of handrails or bars during sitting and standing in the washroom is necessary. Educating self-care strategies to patients such as taking frequent rest breaks while going for long walks, playing, and doing any kind of physical activity. Planning a head of activities is also useful to avoid the stress of rushing to prevent the risk of falls [16].

4.4 Assistive devices and technology

4.4.1 In musculoskeletal management

In order to manage Musculo skeletal issues orthoses play an important role in the prevention of contractures, for joint positioning and standing programmes. In the late ambulatory and early non-ambulatory stages, customized Ankle-foot-orthoses and Knee ankle foot orthoses in accordance with the individual needs and comfort are help full in training standing programmes and assisting in ambulation for therapeutic purposes. Patients with tight long finger flexors should consider resting hand splints.

If contractures are not too severe and restrict positioning, standing aids such as passive standing devices and power standing wheelchairs are taken into consideration in the late ambulatory and early non-ambulatory periods.

4.4.2 In functional training

Functional training includes the assessment of activities of daily living and the need for adaptive equipment or assistive technology.

During the ambulation phase, mostly functional activity is preserved by avoiding a sedentary lifestyle and recommended exercises, and assistive devices are not indicated as they limit certain compensatory movements needed for effective ambulation and they also add difficulty by adding weight to the extremities. Sometimes people need knee ankle foot orthosis with a locked knee to prolong their ambulation phase.

In the early ambulatory stage for long-distance mobility, a lightweight mobility device is necessary. In the late ambulatory stages, an ultra-lightweight manual wheelchair with a solid seat and back rest and footrest are necessary to maintain the spinal symmetry and alignment of the lower extremities.

In the early non-ambulatory stage manual wheelchair with customized seating and recline features is necessary. later in the late non-ambulatory stage, it can be replaced by a powered wheelchair.

As the disease advances, a wheelchair with specialised seating and power positioning components is increasingly required. These components include headrests, solid seats, back and lateral supports, power-adjustable seat height, power-elevating leg rests, pressure-relieving cushions, hip guides, and flip-down knee adductors.

As upper-extremity strength drops in the non-ambulatory phase, rehabilitation assistive technology is required for the evaluation of alternative computer or environment control access, such as a tongue-touch control system, switch scanning, infrared pointing, or eye-gaze selection. Additionally, bathing and bathroom equipment, transfer devices, such as a hydraulic patient lift, ceiling lift (hoist), slide sheets, and environmental control options are all included in the rehabilitation management in the late and non-ambulatory phases of the disease [17].

4.5 Bed mobility exercises

As the progression of diseases, the proper assessment of the musculoskeletal system by the physiotherapist will help to plan for the bed mobility exercise and safe transfer. In the early stage, encourage the subjects to utilize maximal muscle activity and reduce the assisted mobility device utilization. In the late non-ambulatory stages assistive devices are helpful in managing bedridden individuals [21].

4.6 Respiratory muscle training

Baseline pulmonary function tests on all patients with Muscular dystrophy are necessary for the initial phases. Patients should be monitored regularly if they have abnormal baseline pulmonary function test results or any combination of severe proximal weakness, kyphoscoliosis, wheelchair dependence, or comorbid conditions that may affect ventilation.

Subjects with little activity and prolonged sitting or lying positions will lead to decreased chest mobility and diaphragmatic excursion. Respiratory muscles are also involved in the progression of diseases which lead to reduced pulmonary capacity and increased pulmonary complication. Training the subjects initially in the ambulatory phase with Proper positioning and relaxation techniques along with breathing exercises can help them to improve chest mobility and pulmonary capacity [7].

4.7 Swallowing exercise

In muscular dystrophy, the pharyngeal muscles also get involved and lead to swallowing difficulty. A thorough examination is done before the exercise and swallowing exercises are taught to them which will be highly beneficial along with the speech therapist training. Biofeedback stimulation can also be useful to stimulate the pharyngeal muscles to be more active [14].

4.8 Pain management

Muscular dystrophies can cause a variety of pains of varied kinds and intensities. Accurately identifying the reason is necessary for effective pain therapy, which may also include careful team management. There may be a need for pharmaceutical therapies, orthotic intervention, physical therapy, adapted equipment, assistive technology, and postural correction. To put an emphasis on the prevention and management of pain and to maximise pleasant function and movement with the transfer, bathing, and toileting equipment, adaptive equipment and assistive technologies should be used. On motorised wheelchairs and beds, power-positioning components that provide postural support and change, weight transfer, and pressure relief can be used as needed to preserve skin integrity and provide pain relief or prevention (**Table 1**) [22–30].

1. Congenital muscular dystrophy		
	At diagnosis	Evaluate the type of congenital muscular dystrophy, along with other systems of the body Monitor The skeletal system and any other Skeletal abnormalities.
	Early ambulatory stage	Contracture management: Stretching, Orthoses, Standing, Assistive devices. Early intervention exercises and exercises to strengthen the musculature.
	Late ambulatory stage	Therapies to increase range of motion, oedema and swelling:(Hydro kinesiotherapy), Promotion of ADLS, Training of use of assistive technology and Use of customized powered wheelchairs.
	Non-ambulatory stage	Pain management, use of assistive technology.
2. Duchene's Muscular Dystrophy		
	At diagnosis	Multi-disciplinary rehabilitative assessment.
	Early ambulatory stage	Prevention of contracture and deformity: stretching of structures at risk of contracture, orthotic intervention, splinting, casting, positioning and use of equipment, Regular sub maximal, aerobic activity or exercise.
	Late ambulatory stage	Falls, fracture prevention and management with the help of supportive types of equipment for standing and walking.
	Non-ambulatory stage	Use of assistive technology and adaptive equipment and pain management

3. Beckers Muscular dystrophy		
	At diagnosis	Multi-disciplinary rehabilitative assessment.
	Early ambulatory stage	Contracture management: to promote mobility, cramps and fatigue. Exercises such as endurance training help to maintain daily activities, aerobic and resistive training
	Late ambulatory stage	Use of supportive equipment for ambulation
	Non-ambulatory stage	Use of assistive and adaptive devices
4. Emery-Dreyfuss muscular dystrophy		
	At diagnosis	Evaluate the limb muscle weakness in the elbow, neck and spine and early joint contractures.
	Early ambulatory stage	Stretching exercises to promote mobility and prevent contractures
	Late ambulatory stage	Mechanical aids such as canes, walkers and wheelchairs to help with ambulation
	Non-ambulatory stage	Use of assistive and adaptive devices.
5. Limb-girdle Muscular dystrophies		
	At diagnosis	Evaluate the proximal musculature in the shoulder and pelvic girdles and in some cases, involvement of distal muscles is also seen. Evaluation of spinal abnormalities and limb contractures is also a must.
	Early ambulatory stage	Contracture prevention with the help of stretching and splinting orthoses in order to maximise functional ability. Gentle exercise within comfortable limits and the avoidance of prolonged immobility.
	Late ambulatory stage	Fall and fracture prevention strategies, Cardiorespiratory management.
	Non-ambulatory stage	Use of assistive and adaptive equipment
6. Fascio scapula humeral Muscular dystrophy		
	At diagnosis	Evaluate the overhead activities along with Fascial and shoulder girdle muscles and in some cases, it may affect the extraocular, pharyngeal, lingual, abdominal and lower extremities, Hence assessing these sections is also necessary.
	Early ambulatory stage	Flexibility training includes stretching and range of motion exercises, moderate-intensity resistive strengthening exercises moderate-intensity aerobic training programs
	Late ambulatory stage	In the cases where lower extremities are affected use of braces and orthoses for the support of ambulation is required.
	Non-ambulatory stage	Use of assisted powered wheelchairs for ambulation, respiratory and swallowing management with the help of respective professionals.
7. Mayotonic muscular dystrophy		
	At diagnosis	Evaluate cognition and communication, functional activities, and specific patterns of muscles like fascial muscles, neck hand and distal ankle muscles.
	Early ambulatory stage	Exercises such as flexibility, strength training, and cardiovascular and balance training are necessary for children with myotonic dystrophy and should be referred for early intervention exercises to improve fine and motor development, Aquatic therapy and hippotherapy have also proven beneficial.

	Late ambulatory stage	Pain and fatigue management, use of orthotics for gait abnormalities, use of canes, walkers, wheelchairs, and powered mobility devices can be used to allow a person to continue to be safe and independent in mobility
	Non-ambulatory stage	Use of assistive devices and adaptive equipment for continuing their daily activities.
8. Oculopharyngeal Muscular dystrophy		
	At diagnosis	Evaluate muscles of the eye and pharynx muscles and swallowing abilities. In some cases, Fascial muscle weakness, and proximal muscle weakness are also seen.
	Early ambulatory stage	If there is any neuromuscular involvement of lower limbs, contracture management, and exercises to avoid prolonged immobility are necessary.
	Late ambulatory stage	Pain and fatigue management falls and fracture prevention strategies.
	Non-ambulatory stage	Use of assistive and adaptive equipment.
Contribution to quality of life:		
Physiotherapy for muscular dystrophy contributes to assessing gross motor, and fine motor skills, gait ambulation, need for adaptive devices. It helps the individuals in physical well-being by contracture management, and doing exercises and also helps the individuals with the usage of supportive equipment. physiotherapy interventions help muscular dystrophy individuals to do their ADLS Independently which increases their self-efficacy and mental well-being. Pain and fatigue management also play an important role in increasing the quality of life of individuals with muscular dystrophy.		

Table 1.
Physiotherapy interventions for types of muscular dystrophy [22–29].

5. Conclusion

Role of Physiotherapist in proper evaluation and early exercise intervention strategy is more important to maintain the general mobility and thereby improving the physical activity in Muscular dystrophy condition. Based on the different types and severity of the muscular dystrophy, prioritized and patient focused intervention will help to prolong the healthy wellbeing of patient with muscular dystrophy.

Author details

Saina Swathi, Kandhili Chandrasekaran Gayathri and Purushothaman Senthil*
Chettinad School of Physiotherapy, Chettinad Hospital and Research Institute, Chettinad Academy of Research and Education (CARE), Kelambakkam, Tamil Nadu, India

*Address all correspondence to: senthilp101010@gmail.com

IntechOpen

© 2023 The Author(s). Licensee IntechOpen. This chapter is distributed under the terms of the Creative Commons Attribution License (http://creativecommons.org/licenses/by/3.0), which permits unrestricted use, distribution, and reproduction in any medium, provided the original work is properly cited.

References

[1] Emery AE. The muscular dystrophies. Lancet (London, England). 2002;**359**(9307):687-695. DOI: 10.1016/S0140-6736(02)07815-7

[2] Salari N, Fatahi B, Valipour E, Kazeminia M, Fatahian R, Kiaei A, et al. Global prevalence of Duchenne and Becker muscular dystrophy: A systematic review and meta-analysis. Journal of Orthopaedic Surgery and Research. 2022;**17**(1):96. DOI: 10.1186/s13018-022-02996-8

[3] Bell CF, Kurosky SK, Candrilli SD. Muscular dystrophy-related hospitalizations among male pediatric patients in the United States. Hospital Practice (1995). 2015;**43**(3):180-185. DOI: 10.1080/21548331.2015.1033375

[4] Carter JC, Sheehan DW, Prochoroff A, Birnkrant DJ. Muscular d. Clinics in Chest Medicine. 2018;**39**(2):377-389. DOI: 10.1016/j.ccm.2018.01.004

[5] The Lancet. Muscular dystrophy: New treatments, new hopes. Lancet (London, England). 2019;**394**(10213):1966. DOI: 10.1016/S0140-6736(19)32935-6

[6] LaPelusa A, Kentris M. Muscular Dystrophy. Treasure Island, FL: StatPearls Publishing; 2023

[7] Tawil R, Kissel JT, Heatwole C, Pandya S, Gronseth G, Benatar M, et al. Evidence-based guideline summary: Evaluation, diagnosis, and management of facioscapulohumeral muscular dystrophy: Report of the Guideline Development, Dissemination, and Implementation Subcommittee of the American Academy of Neurology and the Practice Issues Review Panel of the American Association of Neuromuscular & Electrodiagnostic Medicine. Neurology. 2015;**85**(4):357-364. DOI: 10.1212/WNL.0000000000001783

[8] Duan D, Goemans N, Takeda SI, Mercuri E, Aartsma-Rus A. Duchenne muscular dystrophy. Nature Reviews. Disease Primers. 2021;**7**(1):13

[9] Thada PK, Bhandari J, Umapathi KK. Becker Muscular Dystrophy. Treasure Island, FL: StatPearls Publishing; 2021

[10] Heller SA, Shih R, Kalra R, Kang PB. Emery-Dreifuss muscular dystrophy. Muscle & Nerve. 2020;**61**(4):436-448

[11] Bushby KM. Diagnostic criteria for the limb-girdle muscular dystrophies: Report of the ENMC Consortium on Limb-Girdle Dystrophies. Neuromuscular Disorders: NMD. 1995;**5**(1):71-74. DOI: 10.1016/0960-8966(93)e0006-g

[12] Narayanaswami P, Weiss M, Selcen D, David W, Raynor E, Carter G, et al. Evidence-based guideline summary: diagnosis and treatment of limb-girdle and distal dystrophies: report of the guideline development subcommittee of the American Academy of Neurology and the practice issues review panel of the American Association of Neuromuscular & Electrodiagnostic Medicine. Neurology. 2014;**83**(16):1453-1463. DOI: 10.1212/WNL.0000000000000892

[13] Johnson NE. Myotonic muscular dystrophies. CONTINUUM: Lifelong Learning in Neurology. 2019;**25**(6):1682-1695

[14] Yamashita S. Recent progress in oculopharyngeal muscular dystrophy. Journal of Clinical Medicine. 2021;**10**(7):1375

[15] Mah JK. Current and emerging treatment strategies for Duchenne muscular dystrophy. Neuropsychiatric Disease and Treatment. 2016;**12**:1795-1807. DOI: 10.2147/NDT.S93873

[16] Birnkrant DJ, Bushby K, Bann CM, Apkon SD, Blackwell A, Brumbaugh D, et al. Diagnosis and management of Duchenne muscular dystrophy, part 1: diagnosis, and neuromuscular, rehabilitation, endocrine, and gastrointestinal and nutritional management. The Lancet. Neurology. 2018;**17**(3):251-267. DOI: 10.1016/S1474-4422(18)30024-3

[17] Bushby K, Finkel R, Birnkrant DJ, Case LE, Clemens PR, Cripe L, et al. Diagnosis and management of Duchenne muscular dystrophy, part 2: implementation of multidisciplinary care. The Lancet. Neurology. 2010;**9**(2):177-189. DOI: 10.1016/S1474-4422(09)70272-8

[18] Birnkrant DJ, Bushby K, Bann CM, Alman BA, Apkon SD, Blackwell A, et al. Diagnosis and management of Duchenne muscular dystrophy, part 2: respiratory, cardiac, bone health, and orthopaedic management. The Lancet. Neurology. 2018;**17**(4):347-361. DOI: 10.1016/S1474-4422(18)30025-5

[19] Green J. Fitness training for clients with muscular dystrophy. Exercise and Fitness, NCHPAD – Building Healthy Inclusive Communities. [Internet] Available from: https://www.nchpad.org/Articles/9/Exercise~and~Fitness

[20] Ashizawa T, Gagnon C, Groh WJ, Gutmann L, Johnson NE, Meola G, et al. Consensus-based care recommendations for adults with myotonic dystrophy type 1. Neurology. Clinical Practice. 2018;**8**(6):507-520. DOI: 10.1212/CPJ.0000000000000531

[21] Zade R, Shende G, Sahu P, Fating T, Deshpande S, Phansopkar P. Rehabilitation in Duchenne muscular dystrophy: A case report. Journal of Pharmaceutical Research International. 2021;**33**(33B):114-120

[22] Angelini C, Marozzo R, Pegoraro V. Current and emerging therapies in Becker muscular dystrophy (BMD). Acta Myologica: Myopathies and Cardiomyopathies: Official Journal of the Mediterranean Society of Myology. 2019;**38**(3):172-179

[23] Lombardo ME, Carraro E, Sancricca C, Armando M, Catteruccia M, Mazzone E, et al. Management of motor rehabilitation in individuals with muscular dystrophies. 1st Consensus Conference report from UILDM – Italian Muscular Dystrophy Association (Rome, January 25-26, 2019). Acta Myologica: Myopathies and Cardiomyopathies: Official Journal of the Mediterranean Society of Myolog. 2021;**40**(2):72-87. DOI: 10.36185/2532-1900-046

[24] Norwood F, de Visser M, Eymard B, Lochmüller H, Bushby K, EFNS Guideline Task Force. EFNS guideline on diagnosis and management of limb girdle muscular dystrophies. European Journal of Neurology. 2007;**14**(12):1305-1312

[25] Thornton CA, Wang E, Carrell EM. Myotonic dystrophy: Approach to therapy. Current Opinion in Genetics & Development. 2017;**44**:135-140. DOI: 10.1016/j.gde.2017.03.007

[26] Trollet C, Boulinguiez A, Roth F, et al. Oculopharyngeal muscular dystrophy. In: Adam MP, Mirzaa GM, Pagon RA, et al., editors. GeneReviews® [Internet]. Seattle (WA): University of Washington, Seattle; 1993-2023; 2001 [Updated 2020 Oct 22]. Available from: https://www.ncbi.nlm.nih.gov/sites/books/NBK1126

[27] Fecek C, Emmady PD. Facioscapulohumeral muscular

dystrophy. In: StatPearls [Internet]. Treasure Island (FL): StatPearls Publishing; 2023 [Updated 2023 Jun 26]. Available from: https://www.ncbi.nlm.nih.gov/books/NBK559028/

[28] Case LE, Apkon SD, Eagle M, Gulyas A, Juel L, Matthews D, et al. Rehabilitation management of the patient with Duchenne muscular dystrophy. Pediatrics. 2018;**142**(Suppl 2):S17-S33. DOI: 10.1542/peds.2018-0333D

[29] Jacques MF, Stockley RC, Onambele-Pearson GL, et al. Quality of life in adults with muscular dystrophy. Health and Quality of Life Outcomes. 2019;**17**:121. DOI: 10.1186/s12955-019-1177-y

[30] Zebracki K, Drotar D. Pain and activity limitations in children with Duchenne or Becker muscular dystrophy. Developmental Medicine and Child Neurology. 2008;**50**(7):546-552

Chapter 6

Role of Applied Physiology in Management of Muscular Dystrophy by Yoga and Meditation

Rituparna Barooah

Abstract

Muscular dystrophies are a group of neuromuscular disorders of genetic origin, Duchene muscular dystrophy being one of the severe forms with no predilection for any ethnicity. The progressive weakness and muscle degeneration culminate in cardiac, respiratory and orthopaedic complications, often accompanied with emotional and psychological involvement. Scope of the introduction of yoga exists at all stages of the disease as an adjunct therapy in prevention of complications, arrest/slowing of progression of the pathophysiology, improvement in the quality of life with better psychosocial adjustment. The science of yoga was developed in ancient India from Eastern Sankhya philosophy in an attempt at establishment of mind–body alignment towards an ideal, intact human physiology. Yoga involves implementation of lifestyle measures aimed at physical, and cognitive development, management of emotions and spiritual conflicts and practicing non-attachment to material and worldly pursuits. Beneficial effects were noted in psychosomatic diseases of non-communicable nature. Practice of yoga in the form of asana (postures), pranayama (breath work), sensory withdrawal (pratyahara), introspection (swadhaya), cultivation of social and individual restraints and practices (yama and niyama) and focused relaxation (dharana and dhyana) has exhibited beneficial physiological change regarding, immunological profile, cardiopulmonary exercise tolerance, posture and equilibrium, sensory acumen, neuromuscular coordination, muscle strength and cognition.

Keywords: Duchene muscular dystrophy, yoga, neuromuscular coordination, physiological effects, muscle strength, asana, pranayama

1. Introduction

Yoga is an ancient Indian technology lifestyle management developed, more than 5000 years ago. It is conglomeration of philosophy positive psychology, emotional intelligence, art and science, all rolled into one package. The science and art of 'living life' has roots in the Eastern Philosophy of Sankhya Yoga. The word yoga is derived from the Sanskrit word 'Yuj' which literally means 'to yoke' or 'to unite'. The three meanings assigned to yoga by scholars are to bind, union and identification with the self and the divine leading to inner peace and freedom. The true perspective of the psychospiritual lifestyle of yoga is to alleviate pain and suffering [1]. Consistent

IntechOpen

practice of the system of physical postures (asana), breathing and mental training with Ayurveda (indigenous native healing practice of India) leads to a higher state of consciousness and awareness of the non-suffering nature of the soul. In the words of Yoga Scholar, George Feuerstein 'yoga therapy is an attempt at integrating traditional yoga concepts and techniques with western medical and psychological knowledge [2]. Yoga therapy aims at alignment of mind and body with a sense of harmony with one's own self and the universe. Practice of yoga therapy is advised in all chronic ailments either as a palliative measure or as complementary therapy [3]. Concept of koshas or layers of existence – five sheaths of physical layer, energy layer, mind, intellect and innermost bliss constituting of gross physical body, subtle body (mental, cognition and emotional and intellect, and innermost layer of the self or the soul) and energy vortices (chakras) are components of yoga and yoga therapy along with diet and nutrition [1]. Chakras are associated with glands and their secretions situated almost along the vertebral column in the midline, namely mooladhara at the base of the spine, swadhisthana, at the level of the genitalia (sacral), manipura or the solar plexus at the level of the navel, anahata chakra at the level of the heart, vishudhi chakra at front of neck, agna chakra in between the eyebrows and sahasrara chakra at the top of the head at the vertex. These are the place where overwhelming emotional feelings are expressed, such as butterflies in stomach, heartache, choking, etc. Yoga includes application of physical postures, breathing techniques, code of conduct, diet, cleansing and detoxifying techniques and deep relaxation techniques, all with total awareness.

Practice of physical posture (yogasanas) causes postural alignments, improves strength, neuromuscular coordination, endurance, balance and flexibility. The breath work (pranayama) is a set of breathing techniques that help to improve the lung capacity and oxygenation of the cells and opens up the chest cavity along with practice of appropriate yogasana. Moreover, the practice of conscious breathing patterns also leads to enhanced perception of body and mind with its thoughts and emotions. Therefore, combined with calming postures and gradual physical stretches (awareness of somatic sensations) with mindful meditation (awareness of thoughts and emotions), continual self-reflection and introspection), yoga transcends mundane life, with conscious inhibition of overthinking and selective and limited energy-consuming distractions. Thus consistent practice of yogic lifestyle with yogic diet and detoxification and purifying techniques increase resilience of the mental turbulence and clutter in the mind is reduced, thoughts are focused on self-care, compassion aimed at seeking harmony with universe and life in general. The autonomic nervous system regains its balance by stimulating the parasympathetic limb whereby relaxation occurs, thus promoting enhanced digestion, blood flow, respiration, regulation of emotion and thoughts [4].

Maharishi Patanjali, the founder of modern yoga describes ashtanga yoga with its eight limbs as a complete set of yogic practice. The eight limbs that were described by him are yama (moral code of conduct), niyamas (personal discipline), asana, pranayama, pratyahara (sensory withdrawal), dharana (one point focused concentration), dhyana (withdrawal from worldly attachments and a state of relaxed concentration on the object of dharana) and samadhi (state of no conflict, absolute acceptance and stilling of turbulence of mind, joy, bliss and freedom). Yama and niyamas are further classified into ahimsa (abstinence from violence), satya (adherence to truth), asteya (non-stealing), brahmacharyya (limitation of worldly attachments) and aparigraha (limitation of needs and wants) [5].

Since yoga is essentially a form of mind-body medicine, consistent and regular practice of yoga lends a positive and promotive outlook to health and life. And to achieve this, all eight limbs of yoga function synergistically to a great extent for a purposeful and meaningful life. Yoga has been classified as a complementary and alternative form of therapy by the National Institute of Health. Yoga therapy mainly relies on four significant principles namely, consideration of the human body as a holistic entity attuned to nature, respect and reverence for individual unique characteristics, healthcare beginning with self-care, compassion and empowerment and lastly cultivation of a positive, accommodating mindset with acceptance [6]. Yoga therapy is particularly appealing as it is devoid of any untoward side effects. Nevertheless, yoga therapy and techniques are best performed and mastered with expert instructors in the field.

2. Therapeutic benefits of yoga and mechanism of action

How does yoga work? Yoga philosophy is founded on self-regulation. Yoga practice functions as a skillset integrating higher and lower brain networks. Self-regulation includes self-monitoring, self-discipline and motivation towards the achievement of the desired goal.

As mentioned earlier, the main therapeutic benefit of yoga is attainment of tranquillity of mind coupled with experience of bliss and joy. A conflict-free mind and a fulfilling sense of well-being even in the face of an incapacitating ailment is what yoga aims for.

There is an increase in self-confidence and efficiency, attentiveness and lowered irritability.

There is also an enhancement of positive outlook, optimism and self-awareness and empowerment with improvement in quality of life.

Inhibition of posterior hypothalamus responsible for sympathetic drive is attenuated with complementary activation of parasympathetic response restoring adapting autonomic reflexes.

This also leads to decrease in anxiety level, heart rate, blood pressure and cardiac output.

Greater prefrontal activity with suppression of limbic subcortical nuclei as in amygdala is reflected by decrease in fear, anger, rage and aggressiveness. Cortical thickness is greater in practitioners of yoga and regular meditators [7].

Stimulation of dopaminergic connections and dopaminergic neurons activate the reward area leading to a sense of fulfilment, pleasure and joy. Mood elevation also follows increase in serotonin levels with concurrent decrease in the levels of monoamine oxidase levels (MAO) [6].

Reduction of aches and pains in muscles and joints reduce with continued practice of yoga as a result of loosening of joints which are exposed to the full range of movement. Blood flow to the joint, capsule, cartilage and muscle increases. Lymphatic circulation is also activated and so are the proprioceptors. Infect, many chronic orthopaedic conditions exhibit a considerable amount of pain reduction [6, 8]. Deep relaxation, gentle stretches, static or dynamic, conscious breathing, visualisation, self-awareness and meditation are techniques to reduce pain.

Blood flow increase with the daily repetitive muscle stretches across the joint and hence, the oxygenation of the tissue and rapid clearing of the metabolites. This leads to increased demand for haemoglobin formation for binding with oxygen and increases tidal volume. With the rapid flow, risk of heart attack and stroke also decreases [6]. Platelet reactivity along with nitrous oxide release potentiates hypocoagulability state following yoga practice. Fibrinogen levels are also found to be decreased and activated partial thromboplastin time and platelet aggregation time increased. Number of blood cells and platelets is also increased. Haemoglobin and haematocrit levels are also increased at the end of the training period [9].

Also, metabolic profile is improved following yoga training and practice. Insulin sensitivity increases, and there is a substantial increase in glucose tolerance and improved lipid profile. Reduced stress perception leads to reduced activation of sympathoadrenal system and HPA axis with resultant reduction in oxidative stress and improved endothelial functions [10].

Since the consistent practice of yogic techniques involve isometric contraction, it leads to increase in skeletal muscle strength of inspiratory and expiratory muscles. There occurs steady and progressive improvement in peak expiratory flow rate (PEFR) and forced expiratory volume FEV1 [11].

Inflammatory markers such as tumour necrosis factor alpha (TNF α) and interleukin 6 (IL-6) are markedly reduced in regular yoga practitioners, making them less prone to inflammatory diseases [12] as compared to age and anthropometric-matched non-practitioners of yoga. Similar observations were recorded in a study with 200 participants over a three-month study period of yoga exposure. Significant increase was observed in levels of anti-inflammatory IL-10 with concurrent decrease in proinflammatory IL-12 levels. Significant increase was observed in the levels of TNF-α, IFN-γ, IL-1β, IL-6 and IL-8 along with an increase in brain-derived nerve growth factor BDNF levels [13, 14].

3. Which type of yoga?

There are many formats of presentation in yoga based on the emphasis of techniques practised. They are karma yoga (emphasis on duty), bhakti yoga (emphasis on surrender and devotion), jnana yoga (knowledge-based), kriya yoga (based on energy modulation), tantra yoga (based on chanting of hymns and prayers) and Patanjali s yoga of eightfold aspects is called raja yoga (royal yoga), a complete package with physical, mental and spiritual aspects of wellbeing.

Hatha yoga refers to another format which emphasises more on the physical aspect, that is, practice of yogasanas and pranayama, cleansing and detoxifying processes. Cleansing and detoxifying consist of fasting and forced vomiting and should be practiced only under expert guidance, and not to be tried without proper evaluation.

Pranayama is made of two words, prana (breath) and ayama (stretching). Pranayama, therefore, consists of a set of breathwork where the pattern of breath (inhalation and exhalation) is stretched and lengthened to the practitioner's capability. Few of the breath work also requires the breath to be held either after inhalation before expelling the air out or following exhalation or before taking the air in. This type of breath work with breath holding is called kumbhaka.

Based on the pattern of emphasis on the phase of respiration, few of the major pranayama are alternate nostril breathing (where inhalation occurs through the nostril through which air was expelled in the previous cycle), bhastrika with active and forceful inhalation and passive exhalation. Kapalbhati is another such technique where the emphasis is on exhalation (forceful and active). Though considered a type of pranayama, kapalbhati is a cleansing technique through breathwork.

Principles for yogasanas can be performed by anyone of any age of ethnicity and culture.

Any posture is an asana when the movements are synchronised with respiratory excursions. The objective of yoga is to cultivate awareness: awareness of the body, mind, emotions, thought, self (purpose and meaning), environment, awareness itself as well as unawareness – Swami Gitananda.

The principles to be followed in practice of yogasanas are

- The movements are slow and steady and focused attention is on the movement.
- Inhalation in each opening movement and exhalation on closing or constricting movement
- Postures must be carried out on both sides. Right-sided movement must be followed with left.
- Each posture is followed with a complementary posture using the opposite muscle group. For example, a forward bend must be followed by a backward bend.
- Yogasana can be done anywhere, in any posture, whether standing, sitting or lying down. Simple yogasanas are possible in wheelchair-bound patients also.
- There is no specific time for yoga. However, yogasanas and pranayamas are best done in the mornings. Meditation is done following the asana and before bedtime.
- There is no dosage or limit for yoga. It can be practiced any number of times up to the capacity and capabilities of the practitioner. Manipulation becomes easier gradually as one progresses through the practice.

Breath is the bridge between body and mind. Pranayama is best practiced early in the mornings, before meal and in open/well-ventilated space in a peaceful surrounding, better still in natural surroundings. Pranayamas are many types though anyone can practice; it is better to be selective according to the time of the day, season and environmental temperature and the affliction or dosha of the subject. Pranayamas are better practiced as standalone performance or after yogasanas. Pranayama or breath regulation practice consists of three steps usually

1. a slow deep inhalation (puraka),
2. long and complete exhalation (rechaka) and
3. kumbhaka which is breath retention, either between inhalation and exhalation (antarkumbhaka) or between exhalation and inhalation (bahirkumbhaka).

Some of the types of pranayamas, which could be beneficial in muscular dystrophy are:

1. The three-stage pranayama which is one of the basic types of pranayamas for practicing breath awareness and increasing the lung function, expansion of the chest cavity and opening of airways. In a comfortable position, normal breaths are taken for a couple of cycles and then with deep inhalation abdominal wall is

pushed outwards. As the inhalation continues, chest is expanded onto the neck region and with raising of the clavicular region and lifting of the shoulders. The reverse occurs in exhalation, first lowering the shoulder and clavicles, followed by gradual expulsion of air from the chest and finally squeezing the abdominal wall to the navel. This is one cycle and such cycles are continued to the capacity and capability of the patient and gradually increased. Continued practice of this deergha pranayama with constant focused attention the breath also relaxes the mind and is very efficient in slowing thought trafficking.

2. Nadishodhana or channel cleaning pranayama is a type of alternate nostril breathing. Right nostril is closed with the right thumb and exhalation is performed through the left nostril following a normal breath. Air is inhaled through the left nostril. Thereafter, the left nostril is closed with the ring finger of the same hand while slowly releasing the thumb on the right nostril for exhalation to occur. The next breath is inhaled through the right nostril and exhaled through the left nostril by lifting the ring finger. This comprises one cycle. Three to six such cycles may be attempted as per the capacity and gradually the number of cycles may be increased. Focus and attention should be on the length of inhalation and exhalation with as less noisily as possible.

3. The nadi-shodhana pranayama may be accompanied by breath holding (retention) after complete inhalation with both nostrils closed when it is termed as anulom vilom, as the subject becomes more familiar with the breathing pattern.

4. Kapalbhati: forceful, active exhalation with pulling of the abdomen towards the navel.

5. Bhastrika: rapid and forceful inhalation and exhalation

Consistent and long-term practice of pranayama and breath regulation help to regulate the vital energies to bring about harmony in autonomic functions [15].

Other significant physiological parameters affected by pranayama are reduction in the heart rate and both systolic and diastolic blood pressure with the practice of slow breathing.

There exists demonstrable evidence of decreased perceived stress scale score with practice of both slow and rapid breathing patterns. Improvement in self-regulation, mood and positivity has been noted. With regular long-term practice of pranayama, enhancement of neurophysiological and psychological function including emotional regulation and processing of emotions ensues [16, 17]. Most often, yogasana, pranayama and meditation are practiced together in a single sitting, in the order of asana, pranayama and meditation. HPA axis and simultaneous activation of neurohumoral also adds to reduction of stress and anxiety and improved quality of sleep by regulating pineal gland function and secretion of melatonin [15].

4. Usefulness and relevance of yoga therapy in Duchene muscular dystrophy

Duchene muscular dystrophy is the most common and severe form of muscular dystrophy culminating in unfortunate premature fatality arising out of cardiorespiratory complications. Breathing exercises can improve the respiratory functions to a great extent.

Hath yoga practice with pranayama especially kapalbhati and yogic breathing can improve lung function as well as increase the strength of the muscles if expiration which is the earliest to be affected. Thus decreasing hospital admission rate and complications [18, 19].

Back pain, osteoarthritis and fibromyalgia also have shown decline in musculoskeletal disorders through gentle yogic postures [20]. Report of improved mobility, respiratory function and quality of life had been documented while on medication [21, 22].

Home-based yoga in Duchene muscular dystrophy has also showed improvement in heart rate variability. The children and parents were taught the exercises for a week. 124 DMD children were assessed in 5 years to 10 years, still ambulatory, with genetically confirmed DMD [23]. The protocol included the practice of gentle muscle stretches and breathing techniques along with other forms of physical therapy and another group with physical therapy alone. Parasympathetic trend showed a rising trend starting during the last 3 months of the study and remained stable for more than 1 year. Although the PT group too showed improvement, it was not long-lasting. Additionally, the children from 5 to 6 years demonstrated a significant earlier and sustained improvement. Strength and mobility were improved. Climbing activity was not much affected. With yoga, physical therapy provides a cardio-respiratory protective effect as well [24].

Studies done on palliative care showed improved quality of sleep, decrease in anxiety and overall improved quality of life with adequate stress management [24]. Emotional mastery and spirituality are two major fallouts achieved through regular practice of pranayama, which is immensely helpful in reducing the added anxiety and apprehension connected to clinical conditions as in Duchene muscular dystrophy imparting a great sense of control and autonomy over one's own life. The reduced autonomic activity and parasympathetic dominant state help to achieve a calmer, peaceful state. These effects are mediated by either dopamine beta-hydroxylase, monoamine oxidase or adrenal steroids.

Yoga has the potential to be an excellent home-based adjunct therapy option offering holistic well-being. Not only muscle strength, flexibility, tone and endurance are increased but also provides emotional stability and positive attitude.

Breathing exercise or pranayamas with activation of muscles of respiration helps to increase the expansion of chest and lung function with considerable decrease in airway obstruction and clearing of the airways. This is well evidenced by electromyography studies that abdominal and oblique muscles are more effectively activated by yogic pranayamas than standard exercises.

Activation of expiratory muscles is much helpful for efficient aeration in patients of DMD.

Sarcopenia and loss of muscle mass are prevented and bone muscle density is also increased. Activities of daily living (ADL) have also been documented to improve. Manual muscle testing (MMT), records increased strength in distal, proximal and axial muscles following home-based yoga programme [25]. The reduction in catecholamine and angiotensin II levels, increased bioavailability of nitrous oxide go a long way to improving the circulation and perfusion of the muscles. In DMD along with anti-inflammatory actions of yoga (lowered IL-6 and C-reactive protein). It had been noticed that fibrosis was also reduced [25].

The programme is also beneficial in causing greater self-care and active interest, participation and involvement in daily activities. Chronic pain is reduced by improved aeration and perfusion, muscle atrophy is avoided causing improved motor function. Muscle strength and balance are certainly improved.

5. Conclusion

Effects of yogic practices have not been studied in much detail as in other non-communicable diseases including cancer of either genetic and hereditary or otherwise [26]. Yoga therapy is a science with a preventive, promotive, curative and palliative approach with not much preparation and precaution and teaches to embrace suffering for the upliftment of the soul [1]. Therefore, there is tremendous scope of application of yoga in afflictions such as in muscular dystrophy. Yoga is a useful tool for coping with stress for immediate caregivers also.

Studies and research on usefulness and implementation of yoga therapy in muscular dystrophies are very minimal, hence we have undertaken to propagate and promote the palliative aspect of yoga therapy.

Acknowledgements

To all my masters from who I learnt the philosophy and techniques of yoga, to the Divine to endow me with an opportunity to be introduced to yoga, to my colleagues and my students for providing opportunity to help propagate the philosophical science of Yoga by way of research and education. Life is a whirlpool of experiences. I owe my gratitude to all who have contributed to my journey into the yogic path, even in the smallest way. I bow in reverence to the guru and the master in all souls in the universe.

Author details

Rituparna Barooah
Physiology, North Eastern Indira Gandhi Regional Institute of Research and Medical Sciences (NEIGRIHMS), Shillong, India

*Address all correspondence to: drrituparnabarooah1@gmail.com

IntechOpen

© 2023 The Author(s). Licensee IntechOpen. This chapter is distributed under the terms of the Creative Commons Attribution License (http://creativecommons.org/licenses/by/3.0), which permits unrestricted use, distribution, and reproduction in any medium, provided the original work is properly cited.

References

[1] Balayogi BA. Principles and methods of yoga therapy notes. In: Yoga Therapy Notes. Pondicherry, South India: International Centre for Yoga Education and Research, & Yoganjali Natyalayam; 2019. pp. 33-39

[2] Karen C. The emerging field of yoga therapy v Ca e S. Hawaii Medical Journal. 2001;**60**(Nov):286-287

[3] Monro R. Yoga therapy. Journal of Bodywork and Movement Therapies. 1997;**1**(4):215-218

[4] Stephens I. Medical yoga therapy. Children. 2017;**4**(2):1-20

[5] Magotra A, Rao MR, Itagi RK, Srinivasan TM. Concept and role of Ashtanga yoga in health promotion wsr to definition of health by World Health Organization. Journal of Ayurveda Integrative Medicine Science. 2019;**4**(03):104-107

[6] Woodyard C. Exploring the therapeutic effects of yoga and its ability to increase quality of life. International Journal of Yoga. 2011;**4**(2):49

[7] Lazar SW, Kerr CE, Wasserman RH, Gray JR, Greve DN, Treadway MT, et al. Meditation experience is associated with increased cortical thickness. Neuroreport. 2005;**16**(17):1893-1897

[8] Büssing A, Ostermann T, Lüdtke R, Michalsen A. Effects of yoga interventions on pain and pain-associated disability: A meta-analysis. Journal of Pain. 2012;**13**:1-9

[9] Bali HK. Yoga-an ancient solution to a modern epidemic. Ready for prime time? Indian Heart Journal. 2013;**65**:132-136

[10] Singh VP, Khandelwal B, Sherpa NT. Psycho-neuro-endocrine-immune mechanisms of action of yoga in type II diabetes. Ancient Science of Life. 2015;**35**(1):12

[11] Mandanmohan JL, Udupa K, Bhavanani AB. Effect of yoga training on handgrip, respiratory pressures and pulmonary function. Indian Journal of Physiology and Pharmacology. 2003;**47**(4):387-392

[12] Vijayaraghava A, Doreswamy V, Narasipur OS, Kunnavil R, Srinivasamurthy N. Effect of yoga practice on levels of inflammatory markers after moderate and strenuous exercise. Journal of Clinical Diagnostic Research. 2015;**9**(6):CC08-CC12

[13] Cahn BR, Goodman MS, Peterson CT, Maturi R, Mills PJ. Yoga, meditation and mind-body health: Increased BDNF, cortisol awakening response, and altered inflammatory marker expression after a 3-month yoga and meditation retreat. Frontiers in Human Neuroscience. 2017;**11**:315

[14] Chen N, Xia X, Qin L, Luo L, Han S, Wang G, et al. Effects of 8-week hatha yoga training on metabolic and inflammatory markers in healthy, female Chinese subjects: A randomized clinical trial. BioMed Research International. 2016;**2016**:5387258

[15] Singh K, Bhargav H, Srinivasan T. Effect of uninostril yoga breathing on brain hemodynamics: A functional near-infrared spectroscopy study. International Journal of Yoga. 2016;**9**(1):12

[16] Novaes MM, Palhano-Fontes F, Onias H, Andrade KC, Lobão-Soares B,

Arruda-Sanchez T, et al. Effects of yoga respiratory practice (Bhastrika pranayama) on anxiety, affect, and brain functional connectivity and activity: A randomized controlled trial. Frontiers in Psychiatry. 2020;**11**(May):1-13

[17] Sengupta P. Health impacts of yoga and pranayama: A state-of-the-art review. International Journal of Preventive Medicine. 2012;**3**(7):444-458

[18] Rodrigues MR, Carvalho CRF, Santaella DF, Lorenzi-Filho G, Marie SKN. Efeitos de exercícios respiratórios de ioga na função pulmonar de pacientes com distrofia muscular de duchenne: Uma análise exploratória. Jornal Brasileiro de Pneumologia. 2014;**40**(2):128-133

[19] Pradnya D, Nalini A, Nagarathna R, Sendhilkumar R, James T, Raju T, et al. Effect of yoga and physiotherapy on pulmonary functions in children with duchenne muscular dystrophy – A comparative study. International Journal of Yoga. 2021;**14**(2):133

[20] Ward L, Stebbings S, Cherkin D, Baxter GD. Yoga for functional ability, pain and psychosocial outcomes in musculoskeletal conditions: A systematic review and meta-analysis. Musculoskeletal Care. 2013;**11**(4):203-217

[21] Telles S, Balkrishna A, Maharana K. Effect of yoga and ayurveda on duchenne muscular dystrophy. Indian Journal of Palliative Care. 2011;**17**:169-170

[22] Raub JA. Psychophysiologic effects of hatha yoga on musculoskeletal and cardiopulmonary function: A literature review. Journal of Alternative and Complementary Medicine. 2002;**8**(6):797-812

[23] Pradnya D, Nalini A, Nagarathna R, Raju T, Sendhilkumar R, Meghana A, et al. Effect of yoga as an add-on therapy in the modulation of heart rate variability in children with duchenne muscular dystrophy. International Journal of Yoga. 2019;**12**(1):55

[24] Deshpande A. Yoga for palliative care. Integrative Medical Research. 2018;**7**(3):211-213

[25] Saud A, Abbasi M, Merris H, Parth P, Jones XM, Aggarwal R, et al. Harnessing the benefits of yoga for myositis, muscle dystrophies, and other musculoskeletal disorders. Clinical Rheumatology. 2022;**41**:3285-3297

[26] Venditti S, Verdone L, Reale A, Vetriani V, Caserta M, Zampieri M. Molecules of silence: Effects of meditation on gene expression and epigenetics. Frontiers in Psychology. 2020;**11**:1767